TRANSFORMATIONAL
NLP

TRANSFORMATIONAL
NLP

The spiritual approach to
harnessing the power of
Neuro-Linguistic Programming

CISSI WILLIAMS

WATKINS PUBLISHING
LONDON

This edition first published in the UK and USA 2012 by
Watkins Publishing, Sixth Floor, Castle House,
75–76 Wells Street, London W1T 3QH

1 3 5 7 9 10 8 6 4 2

Designed and typeset by Basement Press, Glaisdale

Printed and bound in China

British Library Cataloguing-in-Publication Data Available
Library of Congress Cataloging-in-Publication Data Available

ISBN: 978-1-780-28-122-3

www.watkinspublishing.co.uk

Distributed in the USA and Canada by Sterling Publishing Co., Inc.
387 Park Avenue South, New York, NY 10016-8810

For information about custom editions, special sales, premium and corporate
purchases, please contact Sterling Special Sales Department at 800-805-5489 or
specialsales@sterlingpub.co.uk

This book is dedicated to my beautiful
daughters Erika and Natasha.
May you always know how amazing you are
and that you are meant to manifest all your dreams.
Just have the courage to follow your heart,
take inspired action, have faith and relax
in the knowledge that when the time is right,
your dreams will indeed come true.

About the author

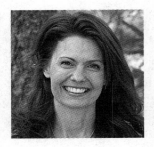 Cissi Williams moved to Sigtuna, Sweden in 2007, where she now lives with her husband and their two daughters, three cats, a Bernese mountain dog and two rabbits.

She offers training in Transformational NLP and Transformational Break-Through Coaching, as well as running personal and spiritual development courses. She treats patients and clients from her and her husband's clinic in Sigtuna, and regularly lectures and holds seminars in Sweden and in the UK.

Together with her husband, she founded the Swedish magazine *Inspire – A Body, Mind and Spirit Guide to Well-Being* with the intention of inspiring others to connect with their own inner healing power and innate well-being, enabling a deep healing of body and mind. She is passionate about sharing with others the tools for connecting with the power within us, enabling us to heal ourselves and our lives, and fulfil our dreams.

If you want to find out more please visit www.nordiclightinstitute.com or www.inspiremagazine.eu

Contents

Acknowledgments

I want to thank my wonderful husband, Alan, and our two precious daughters, Erika and Natasha. I am truly blessed to have you in my life and just being with you is the best gift ever. With you I am able to experience such deep love and happiness it takes my breath away.

I want to thank my dad, who is now in heaven. Thanks to you I was put on this path of healing and you are one of my greatest teachers.

I also want to thank Sandra Rigby, my editor at Watkins Publishing, who contacted me to see if I wanted to write a book about how to use Transformational NLP with a spiritual approach, and a big thank you to editor Jo Godfrey Wood, who had suggested my name to Sandra. To me, it is a miracle how this book came about. Thank you – and also to Fiona Robertson – for being my editing angels!

I want to give a big thank you to my lovely friend Karrin Lawrence, NLP Trainer, who has graced this book and my life with her wisdom and insights. You are such a wonderful friend and I am so glad for that day, many years ago, when your back pain caused you to seek me out for an osteopathy appointment.

I want to thank Adrian Bradshaw-Jones, amazing coach and Master Practitioner of NLP who has, with his extraordinary creativity and insight, illustrated Higher-Self Healing, Parts Integration and Drop Down Through in this book. Thank you!

I also want to thank Rob Purfield and Debbie Jenkins, both NLP Trainers. You were the first to give me feedback on this manuscript. Thank you for your wise insights and wisdom!

I want to thank all my patients, clients and students, who have all made this book possible; thanks to everything they have taught me.

A special thank you to everyone who has loved me and supported me throughout the years: my mum, my sister Jessica, Eva (thank you for being there as my best friend during our whole childhood and for all our wonderful travels together. Our trek in Nepal will always be a magical memory), Almira and Sasha.

I want to thank all my teachers, such as those at the British College of Osteopathy and Naturopathy (now British College of Osteopathic Medicine), as well as David Shepherd, Master Trainer of NLP, John Grinder, co-founder of NLP, Carmen Bostic St Clair, co-developer of NLP, Michael Carroll, Master Trainer of NLP, and all other teachers of spiritual wisdom who have lit up the way for me to follow: Neale Donald Walsch, Eckhart Tolle, Paramahansa Yogananda, Louise Hay, Marianne Williamson, Caroline Myss, Sanya Roman, Gerald Jampolsky, Abraham-Hicks, Lama Surya Das, Wayne Dyer, Tony Robbins, Deepak Chopra, Brandon Bays, Doreen Virtue, Barbara Brennan, Shakti Gawain, Alberto Villoldo, Gregg Braden, Denise Linn, Byron Katie, Sonia Choquette and many, many more.

And finally I want to thank all our friends in Sigtuna, who have made the dark winters in Sweden a little bit more bearable for my British husband (and for me)! You know who you are and I thank you from the bottom of my heart.

PART 1

Introduction to the Magical World of Transformational NLP

Introduction

Transformational NLP as a tool for healing with the Spirit

This book is not just about Neuro-Linguistic Programming (popularly known as NLP); it is about how you can use it as a magical transformational tool, enabling you to heal any area of your life by harnessing the power and wisdom of a greater force – a force I term the Spirit. You may wish to call this power by some other name that is meaningful for you, such as God, Divine Force or Higher Power – the term itself is not important. The key point is that this book will show you how to access a power above and beyond your ego self to allow deep inner healing to take place. My experience as both an NLP coach and therapist has shown me that profound growth can occur when we access wisdom and love from our Spirit, which is then able to flow into our minds and bodies. It is the Spirit that provides us with our life force. By using NLP as a tool to tap into this divine life force you will achieve amazing results.

My passion is to help others empower themselves. This has led me to study a variety of disciplines: osteopathy, cranial osteopathy, naturopathy, NLP, as well as many other sources of wisdom including meditation, visualization, shamanism and prayer. There are many paths leading to the attainment of health, happiness and wisdom. For me NLP is just one of a number of tools that you can use. The key to its effectiveness is how you use it and your intent in using it.

NLP has become a very popular technique for self-help and personal empowerment as it enables people to better understand how their ways of thinking and feeling create their daily experience; it shows us how we can change our habitual ways of behaving, thereby giving us more choices for how we want to "be" in our lives.

NLP became world famous through life coach Tony Robbins and hypnotist Paul McKenna. Both have shown how NLP can quickly and effectively change a person's thinking and behaviour for the better. The discipline is also used widely in the business community as it helps to improve understanding of others, as well as helping to enhance communication with each other.

I was first drawn to NLP when I noticed, through my work as an osteopath, that I could quickly "feel" people's emotions in different parts of their bodies. I realized that just working on them physically would not be the quickest and most efficient way of releasing these emotional imbalances. I understood that many of these negative emotions had originally been caused by negative ways of thinking and past negative experiences. Once I had learnt NLP, I had a truly powerful tool for helping my patients to release the emotional pain that had been held in their bodies – quickly and effectively, in an exquisite way. As I continued to use NLP in my work with patients and coaching clients, I changed what I had been taught by tapping into my own spiritual understanding of how to facilitate healing of the body and mind. This was never a conscious act – it just happened. I was not fully aware of just how different my approach was until my friend Karrin Lawrence met up with me one day after she had finished her NLP Master Practitioner Training with David Shepherd. David is a Master Trainer of NLP and one of the most respected trainers in the UK and I had completed the same training some years previously. I started to work with Karrin using my new approach to NLP. She asked me afterwards:

"What was that you did?"

"It was NLP," I said.

"No, it wasn't. You did something different," Karrin replied.

It seemed that Karrin had healed in a way that went "beyond" the normal workings of NLP.

Karrin encouraged me to develop a course based on these modified techniques, combined with my spiritual knowledge. This is how the course *Transform Your Life – Learn the Tools for Creating Your Dream Life* came into being and this course forms the basis for the material in this book. It was a wonderful experience to see the other course participants take each other through this deeply transformational process. They had no prior training and yet within just a few days they had been able to shed many layers of negativity and connect more fully with the extraordinary wisdom, love and light that resides within each and every one of us.

So what was the basis of the spiritual understanding that I had tapped into naturally?

I had been on a spiritual path since 1992, when I found myself in the depths of a deep depression. I was 24 years of age and I felt seriously suicidal. I had suffered a difficult childhood with a mentally and emotionally ill father and this resulted in a volatile and at times abusive home environment. But this was nothing compared to the emotional abuse to which I had been subjecting myself after I had left home. I had been truly vicious toward myself and this poison had spilled out into my relationships with others.

Then one night I dreamed I saw myself hanging dead in my room in London. When I woke up in the morning I realized that I needed help … and fast. I prayed to a power greater than myself – I prayed to the universe for guidance. I knew that I needed to make drastic changes, but I had no idea how. I just knew that the problem was *me*; it wasn't my childhood or my father, it wasn't even my depression – that was just the expression of the hatred I felt for myself. I knew that I couldn't continue hating myself or I might, indeed, soon be hanging from my ceiling, but I didn't know where to start. As I prayed for a miracle to happen, I felt as if a burden had been lifted. Then I waited. I don't know what I was expecting, but I thought that somehow all the answers would be revealed to me straightaway. Nothing happened, but then I received a spontaneous flash of insight that I should go home to Stockholm; so that is what I did.

The next day I was walking down the streets of my beautiful home town and I suddenly found myself standing outside a bookshop I had never seen before. I went in and immediately felt drawn to three books: *The Power is Within You* by Louise Hay, *Love is the Answer* by Gerald Jampolsky and *Creative Visualization* by Shakti Gawain. I remember sitting in the shop reading these books and realizing that this was what I had prayed for – a way for me to change. These books became my first steps toward healing. During the following few months I read hundreds of books on personal and spiritual development and listened to countless meditation tapes. As I read and meditated my depression lifted. At first it eased only while I was actually reading or meditating, but within a few weeks the effect lasted for several hours. Through meditation I calmed and balanced my mind and in the process neutralized and stilled my emotions. Within six weeks my depression had totally disappeared.

During the autumn of 1992 I realized that I wanted to work in the field of health and healing. I felt drawn to study osteopathy and a year after I'd hit the lowest point of my depression I started a four-year university degree at the British College of Osteopathic Medicine. I became a fully qualified osteopath and naturopath in 1997.

During my osteopathic training I continued to meditate and read spiritual books and I participated in various workshops on personal and spiritual development. I have been greatly influenced by the teachings in *A Course in Miracles* (Foundation for Inner Peace), as well as by the work of authors such as Caroline Myss, Neale Donald Walsch, Eckhart Tolle, Byron Katie, Lama Surya Das, Paramahansa Yogananda, Abraham-Hicks, Denise Linn, Alberto Villoldo, Marianne Williamson, Brian Weiss, Gregg Braden, Wayne Dyer and Gary Zukav, among many others. I had also travelled extensively around Asia and spent a long time in India and Nepal, where I was introduced to yoga and meditation. All these experiences convinced me of the importance of the Spirit in our lives.

I believe we are divine, spiritual beings, in a physical body. The pain we experience in our lives is because we have forgotten who we truly are – that we are the light, we are love, we are an expression of divinity. To heal our pain we have to connect again with this eternal truth. The pain is just an illusion, albeit a very persistent one. However, it is still an illusion, consisting of darkness, and the moment you shine your higher conscious awareness on to it, it disappears. It's the same as when you light a candle in a dark room; the old darkness disappears and instead a beautiful light shines forth.

The key is to find the *structure* of the illusion, of this darkness, and then guide your higher consciousness toward a deep understanding of it. When you do this "magic" happens – a profound transformation takes place, from darkness to light. You begin to shine ever more brightly, ever more strongly.

Your divine light is able to flow ever more freely through you and out into the world.

In my model of the world NLP is a great tool – an exquisite tool. It allows me to diagnose and analyze the structure of a person's internal universe, the structure of their inner darkness that, in turn, is causing problems for their health and in their emotional life. However, to enable a deep healing to take place, I believe you have to connect with a much higher presence, a higher spiritual awareness. It is this higher awareness that provides the wisdom, insights and power that cause personal transformation and healing to take place – the transformation from darkness to light, from negativity to positivity, from fear to love. My intention when I use Transformational NLP is to help free our human consciousness from fear and pain and instead connect more fully with our divine consciousness, while still being anchored fully in the present moment. In this way we are able to have the experience of being in this everyday world of problems and challenges and yet also be aware of the possibility of existing in peace and calmness beyond it.

My special passion and goal in life is to help all individuals evolve to this point of awareness and wisdom. If you feel a calling for this as well, this book will give you some great tools and insights to help you on your path.

How to use this book

The book starts at beginner level, explaining the basic concepts of NLP and then moves on to exploring the principles of Transformational NLP. I cover how to become a "magician" using the power of linguistics. This is the foundation of my Transformational NLP course and I explain various techniques and processes that can be used for healing your inner self, your mind and your life.

The deeply healing and transformational part of this book is introduced in Parts 4 and 5, where you will learn how to develop wisdom and increase your spiritual energy. You will also learn how to heal with your Spirit through the Transformational NLP Break-Through Healing Session (see pages 188–220). This is a very intense and incredibly spiritually cleansing process and you need to allocate at least six or seven hours to the whole process. However, the time and energy you invest in it will be returned to you a hundredfold. You will heal at a deep level by shedding layers of negativity and darkness and by doing this you will connect more fully with your inner light, love and divine potential.

This book also contains coaching sections for those who want to learn how to apply these processes and insights with clients. You can find these sections at the end of various Transformational NLP techniques and they are also found in Part 6 Additional Information for Coaches (pages 222–60). Many of the exercises and techniques are recorded on the audio download available at www.nordiclightinstitute. com. In this way you can just relax and let me guide and coach you on this truly healing and transformational journey.

Perhaps you have picked up this book because you want to find different tools and techniques for developing yourself personally and spiritually, or maybe you are already studying NLP and coaching, or are already using it in your working life. Whatever the reason, this book will help you to develop the skills, linguistic tools and wisdom to enable you to transform the way you think and how you perceive the world you live in. You will learn how to access a higher, divine wisdom that resides within you.

What is important to remember, though, is that these skills, tools and techniques are just that – skills, tools and techniques. They are rather like money. Money is just money – it is neither good nor bad, just a type of energy. It is how you use that energy that determines whether it results in something positive or negative. It is the same with anything in life, including the processes presented in this book. These techniques are very powerful and I strongly urge you to only use them with positive intent, both for yourself and everyone with whom you are connected. When you practise them with positive intent you will find that deep healing and transformation take place, often far more rapidly than you would have thought possible.

I hope and trust that this journey into Transformational NLP will prove as rewarding for you as it has for me and my many clients and students around the world. Enjoy!

PART 2

Transformational NLP and Healing with the Spirit

Chapter 1
A Quick Introduction to NLP

What is Transformational NLP?

Well, answering that is as easy as answering the question, "What is the meaning of life?" You will get different responses – it all depends who you ask.

Let me first ask a few questions:

- Would you like to learn how you can live a life where *you* decide *who* you want to be and *how* you want to behave?
- Would you like to find out how you can choose to empower yourself and connect with your inner positive resources, whenever you need to?
- Would you like to be in control of your mind instead of your mind controlling you and your life?
- Would you like to learn how to follow your inner guidance and take steps to create the life you want to lead, despite inner worry and doubt nagging at you?
- Do you want to be able to listen to your Spirit guiding you and learn processes that can enable you to tap more easily into its amazing wisdom?

Well, if you are anything like me, then you may have answered "Yes" to some, or perhaps all, of these questions. It was my vision of learning how to be the most authentic version of "me" that I could possibly be, and my thirst for learning about the power of the mind and Spirit that eventually led me to study the art and science of NLP – Neuro-Linguistic Programming.

I realized that NLP is about freedom – freedom to be the best that I can possibly be, to live my life to the full, to be happy and fulfilled, whatever life brings me, and to be able to choose who I want to be.

According to NLP we can all learn how to change our thoughts, behaviours and feelings and in this way take back control over our lives, so that we can live the life we want to live and be the person we want to be. But how is this possible and what is NLP?

NLP is a collection of techniques, models and processes for personal development, effective communication, changing unwanted behaviours, letting go of limiting decisions and destructive strategies, and healing old negative emotions. NLP is the study of how the brain works, and as such it can be used highly effectively for emotional, mental and physical healing. NLP techniques enable you to tap into the inherent wisdom, knowledge and healing within the Unconscious Mind (which comprises about 90 per cent of your brain capacity), while allowing the Conscious Mind (the logical, thinking, rational part of the mind, using only about 10 per cent of the brain's capacity) to be completely aware of what is happening. So how is this possible? Before exploring that, let us first discuss the origins of NLP.

The history of NLP

Two exceptional men, John Grinder and Richard Bandler, originally founded NLP in the 1970s. Bandler was enrolled as a young psychology student at the University of California, Santa Cruz, in 1970, and Grinder was an associate professor of linguistics at the same university. Bandler visited Grinder several times to invite him to come along to a session he was holding on Gestalt Therapy, wanting him to analyze the linguistics used. The first few times, Grinder said no, but eventually he relented and went along and this was the start of a very fruitful collaboration. Soon the two men were using Grinder's linguistics to pursue Bandler's interest in the work of Fritz Perls (the founder of Gestalt Therapy).

They continued to develop NLP through asking themselves the following question, "What is it that distinguishes people who do something with extraordinary elegance and outstanding perfection from people who do not?"

Bandler and Grinder decided to seek the answer by studying the work of three renowned therapists who had achieved extraordinary results with their patients and who were all masters of communication. They studied Milton Erickson (a psychotherapist and hypnotherapist), Virginia Satir (a family therapist) and Fritz Perls with a view to finding out what it was that distinguished them from others in those fields.

By studying how these world-renowned therapists and communication experts achieved their outstanding results, Bandler and Grinder managed to extract the key to their success. They wrote down *exactly* what it was that these experts did and managed to discover the strategies, linguistics, processes and techniques that made their work unique. Then Bandler and Grinder tried to see if they, too, could achieve the same sorts of results using the same strategies, linguistics, processes and techniques. After a short time they succeeded. The next step was to teach what they had learned to others, so that they, too, could achieve the same. Bandler and Grinder discovered that this was possible – and NLP was born.

Let us begin to explore NLP

NLP is often described as an attitude and a methodology that leaves a trail of techniques in its wake. The attitude is a sense of curiosity, which enables you to discover new ways of thinking, while the methodology is a toolbox of techniques, designed to create maximum, specific, positive changes and results, allowing you to live the life of your dreams and experience well-being on all levels. It does all this by letting you take charge of the most wonderful computer ever created – your brain.

A definition of NLP

- **Neuro** – this refers to the nervous system and NLP is based on the idea that we experience our reality through our five senses: Visual, Auditory, Kinaesthetic (proprioceptive [our positions in space] and meta [our internal feelings]), Olfactory (smell) and Gustatory (taste). This is outside information streaming in through our five senses, which we then translate into thought processes.

- **Linguistic** – this is how we represent, order and sequence the neural information into models and strategies through language and other non-verbal systems – pictures, sounds, feelings, tastes, smells and self-talk.
- **Programming** – this is the organization of the sensory representations into patterns, to achieve specific outcomes. Personal programming consists of internal processes and strategies (thinking and behaviour patterns). You have a strategy (an order and sequence of specific thoughts) that leads to a particular behaviour for everything you do, whether this is cooking, learning, playing, making decisions, arguing with a loved one, making up with a loved one, going on a date, studying and all the other activities that make up your life.

The map is not the territory

One of the presuppositions (a thought that you act upon as if it is true, although you know it is not always true; it just helps you to find more resources within yourself) in NLP is that *the map is not the territory*. This means that everyone has their own inner screening systems, through which they filter their experiences. These systems affect how we experience our personal inner map of our reality. Every day we move through familiar territories and experiences, but, because we all have different inner screening systems and different inner maps, we all also have different experiences from one another. You and your neighbour will experience the area you live in differently; you and your siblings will have different perceptions of your parents and you and your colleague will have different perceptions about your work environment. We even change our own perception of a certain area or situation depending upon whether we change our inner screening systems and inner map.

We never experience reality as it is

As human beings we can never experience reality as it actually is, since we have to experience it through our five senses and our senses are limited in how much information they can receive. So the information streaming in from the outside world is already limited by our senses. Despite this around two million "bits" of information stream through our senses into our nervous system. To ensure that we are not overwhelmed by this stream, the Unconscious Mind screens out most of it and only five to nine "chunks" (larger than a bit, see page 26) of information reach the Conscious Mind. This figure varies, but a significantly smaller portion of information reaches the Conscious Mind compared to the portion of information reaching the Unconscious Mind.

This inner screening system is our inner map of reality. This is why we don't react to reality, only to our perception of it. We communicate our outer experience to ourselves by translating it into an inner experience through our own physiological reaction – the inner pictures we have, the sounds we hear, as well as the emotions stimulated within. All of this is a neurological interpretation of the experience. We also interpret the experience linguistically through the words we choose when we talk to ourselves. These interpretations form the inner map of our reality.

We all have our own reality of the world around us and this is based upon which type of neuro-linguistic inner map we have formed. This map decides how we interpret an outer experience, how we react to what is happening around us and which meaning we attach to our behaviours and experiences. *We never experience reality as it is, but how we are.* This is why it is usually never outer reality that limits us and causes us problems, but our inner reality, our inner maps and screening systems, which either help us to be happy in life or cause us to feel pain and unhappiness. The information that is filtered through the brain and how it *translates* it affect how we experience life, which in turn influences our behaviour.

Imprints

The inner map or inner screening system consists of our values and decisions about ourselves and others, as well as our early experiences, especially those that in NLP language are called "imprints". An imprint is a memory that was formed at an early age and creates a root thought, which can be either limiting or else resourceful and empowering. Put simply, it is either negative or positive. A negative imprint can give rise to some of our Limiting Thoughts and Limiting Decisions, which can be very unhealthy and damage our ability to live an authentic, happy life. When we have a negative imprint we unconsciously draw negative experiences to us, that mirror the original event that caused the imprint. Imprints affect how we view our reality and when some are negative we tend to view ourselves, others and our reality through negative inner-screening systems. This causes us to experience our reality even more negatively, which affects our ability to deal with difficult situations.

Changing the inner screening system

Using NLP you can change your inner screening systems and maps. This can help you to let go of inner blocks and Negative Thought patterns, which may have stopped you from healing your body, mind, relationships and life. One of the biggest obstacles to healing is your own inability to *believe* in your own inner healing power. If you do not believe that you are going to get better, then you will not take the necessary steps and actions.

In NLP you first work to identify the *structure* of what is causing a problem, such as Negative Thought patterns, Limiting Beliefs and Problem Strategies that exist within the Unconscious Mind. Then NLP uses a variety of processes and techniques to change these Negative Thought patterns and Limiting Beliefs into Positive Thought patterns and resourceful and empowering beliefs instead. This causes the inner screening system and inner maps to change and so your own perception of your reality changes, too.

We all have different inner maps and inner screening systems for different areas of our lives, such as relationships, family, work, personal development, spiritual development and health. As a simple guide, you can say that in those areas that are working well for you in your life you will have positive inner screening systems and positive inner maps, while those areas that are not working so well will contain negative inner screening systems and a negative inner map, weakening your ability to have positive experiences in those areas. Fortunately, your inner screening systems can be changed easily, quickly and effectively, as long as you are willing to take responsibility for your own thoughts, feelings and behaviours. The techniques in this book will enable you to do that.

A personal story of experiencing NLP

What has my own experience of NLP been? My first contact with it was through a friend, Alastair, who had just started training in NLP and wanted to test his new skills on his friends. One evening, during conversation, it came to light that I was very angry and sad about my father. Alastair wondered if I wanted to release these feelings and I enthusiastically said, "Yes". A few minutes later I found myself deep in a trance, although fully aware of what was going on. Alastair got me to go through different mental processes, which I thought were fascinating, new, though somewhat strange. An hour and a half later we had finished and I forgot all about it. A few months later I flew home to Sweden to visit my family. I intended to see my father, which I did and for the first time ever I saw him as the person he truly was and not as the person I thought he was – my inner screening systems had totally changed. Now I saw him as another human being and not as the father I had experienced him to be. I accepted him as he was. All I could feel in his presence was enormous love and gratitude that he was in my life – completely new for me. Previously, whenever I was with him, I had always felt a mixture of love, fear, anger, frustration, anxiety, sorrow and sadness. But this was not the case this time. I didn't actually realize how much I had changed then and there, and it was not until I was on the plane back to London that it suddenly occurred to me and I thought, "Wow! I didn't react in my old way! I was different within myself in Dad's presence."

I then realized that ever since Alastair had coached me in NLP I had stopped thinking about my father negatively. I felt an enormous freedom and happiness within, and during the flight I decided that I would train in NLP so that I could help others solve conflicts and problems in this gracious and effective way. When I met my husband at Heathrow I told him all about it and he agreed that I should do the training. We were worried about being able to afford it, but I knew that I had to do it.

A few months later I became pregnant and realized that I had to do the training quickly, otherwise it would be several years before I got the chance again. So we released some of the equity from our house so that I could pay for the training and I promised myself that I would somehow pay it back before I gave birth to our baby. On the last day of my Master Practitioner training, when I was 35 weeks pregnant, I set as a goal that I would see four Break-Through clients before I gave birth, but I did not really know how this was going to happen.

When I got home there were four phone messages waiting – all from people who wanted to come for a Break-Through session, and I did the last of these a week before our daughter was born. These sessions made me realize that this was what I was meant to do. And the money I received for these four sessions was the exact amount we had released from our equity.

NLP looks to the highest potential

So how was all of this possible? For me, what NLP taught was the art of asking intelligent questions – the more intelligent the question, the more intelligent the answer. NLP uses meaningful and effective linguistics, which can go deeply into the specific details of our experience and *how* we think, as well as finding the highest intention and purpose as to why we do what we do.

In NLP you always look to the highest potential in the individual. This is vital because it acknowledges that we all have the ability within ourselves to change. NLP does not think of a problem as being set in stone. Instead it sees it as a strategy, a certain way of thinking and acting that causes us to get stuck with a negative pattern. With this way of viewing a problem there is no such thing as a *big* problem or a *little* problem; they are all different problems with different strategies and they can *all* be changed. This does not have to be a lengthy process. NLP has become a successful technique because it enables the individual to change quickly and effectively without suffering any side effects. The change occurs ethically and organically because it is the person's own Unconscious Mind that finds all the positive resources, insights and learnings needed to heal the old problem, until it has completely disappeared.

The only thing NLP requires of you is that you are willing to get to know yourself better and that you have the ability and willingness to think differently from your usual way. I have never met anyone who could not allow NLP to help them find more freedom and positive inner resources. Even my children (eight and 13 years old) use NLP naturally, especially in their communication with others (their dad doesn't stand a chance!). It is quite delightful to hear your child use an NLP linguistic technique on you, for example, "So Mummy, can we play a game now or maybe even quicker than that?" (see pages 129–34 for an explanation of the Milton Model double-bind linguistic pattern).

How does NLP work?

NLP works by allowing you to take charge of your brain, by allowing you to run your own neurology, rather than letting your neurology run you. It has a multitude of techniques and tools enabling you to do that, but let me give you a few examples. Say you always react in a certain way in a certain context, so that you have built up a neurology that you fire off as a reaction every time you find yourself in this context. For instance, as soon as a particular person looks at you in a certain way you feel anxious, or as soon as you are speaking in front of an audience you panic, or whenever your mother uses a certain tone of voice you feel bad. NLP allows you to change your reaction in this context, thereby giving you more *choice* about how you want to respond. Remember: NLP is about freedom – freedom to *choose* how you want to be.

Tapping into language

NLP taps into the language your brain uses. Let's try an experiment. Just for a moment think of someone you really love; someone you are really fond of. Picture them in your mind and notice where that picture is located. Is it up, down, left, right, far or near? Then clear the "screen" and think of someone you really dislike; someone you like least in the whole world. Notice where that picture is located. Is it up, down, left, right, far or near?

Are the two locations different? I guess that they are. Now move the picture of the person you dislike to the location of the person you love. Notice whether it makes you feel differently about the person. For some people, it may not even have been possible to move the picture, because the Unconscious Mind was not OK with you liking this person. So you can see that your brain stores information about someone you love and someone you dislike in different ways and puts this in different locations. The brain also stores everything else in a unique way by using finer visual distinctions, such as location, and also finer auditory and kinaesthetic distinctions (we will explore this in detail in the section about submodalities, see pages 64–85). As an NLP coach, knowing the finer distinctions about how someone stores their information can allow you to change how they represent something to themselves, which will change the meaning of their internal representation.

Correlation with ancient wisdom

NLP teaches us that we don't actually respond to reality, but rather to our own interpretation of it. This is the same as what all esoteric teachings tell us. Quantum physics teaches us that nothing exists until we observe it and that everything we observe is affected by the observer. This means that the world we live in is experienced the way it is because of how we *interpret* it.

NLP is concerned with uncovering the *structure* of how you perceive your reality and then helping you to change it so that it becomes enriching and helpful to you. NLP is about freedom – freedom from being controlled by your mind, and instead being in charge of how you use it. Many other traditions and systems of knowledge tell us this. Buddha taught us how to be free from attachments by learning to simply observe our experience without being attached to pleasure or pain – just observing the sensation and realizing that everything passes in time. By practising this you start to learn to control your mind instead of letting it control you and thereby your emotions. NLP helps you to release yourself from addictions (seeking too much pleasure) and helps you to become neutral about painful past experiences (avoiding pain).

In shamanistic traditions you find imprints in the energy field and then use a variety of techniques to erase this imprint. Often imprints are linked to an event that happened a long time ago, in which the person might have made a "soul contract" (a deeply held limiting belief) in order to feel safe. Often these contracts are unpleasant and negative, but with shamanistic treatments you can erase the imprint, fill it with light, and re-negotiate the old contract into a new, positive one instead. In NLP we also work with imprints (we diagnose them in NLP as Problem Strategies, Negative Emotions, Limiting Beliefs and so on) and soul contracts and we help to erase these by taking the client through processes where they change their *thinking* concerning the initial event, which also changes their physiological and emotional charge concerning it – and we guide them to find all the Positive Learnings from it (which is similar to re-negotiating a soul contract into a positive contract). To put it simply, we guide the client to transform negativity into positivity and darkness into light.

In esoteric Christianity you search for the Christ within – the light within. You go deep within to find yourself, to find God within, to find love within. Many of the NLP techniques take you on a journey deep within your inner essence, where you reach a place of complete love, light and happiness.

Up until now, only a few NLP trainers have explored NLP and spirituality in their writing. Robert Dilts wrote *Tools of the Spirit* and he co-authored *The Hero's Journey* with Stephen Gilligan. Tad James introduced some spiritual concepts into the world of NLP because of his deep interest in the ancient Hawaiian spiritual tradition of Huna.

Presuppositions of NLP

The presuppositions of NLP are quite well known. A presupposition is a belief you choose to have, which you know may not be true. However, you act *as if* it is true, in order to help it empower you.

- **Respect other people's Model of the World.**
  We all have a unique Model of the World. This means that we have unique inner filters and screening systems, unique inner maps. It is important to remember that we are all different and unique. My Model of the World may not be the same as yours.

- **People respond to their Model of the World, not to reality.**

  This means that people respond to their inner filters, not what is actually happening. In other words, you never experience the event as *it is* – you experience the event as *you are*.

- **People are *not* their behaviour.**

  This means that we are all so much more than our behaviour. As Martin Luther King Jr so famously said, "I am talking about a type of love, which will cause you to love the person who does the evil deed while hating the deed that the person does."

- **All behaviour has a positive intention.**

  All our behaviour always has a positive intention, even if it sometimes does not appear that way. Remember, this is only a presupposition, so is not necessarily true, but when we act as if it *were* true it helps to empower us, because we can find the positive in any situation and *choose* how we want to respond, rather than just reacting. For example, if my friend snaps at me for no apparent reason, but I believe that she has a positive intention, it is easier for me to look at her behaviour from a higher perspective and then perhaps see that she is snapping because she is stressed – that it has nothing to do with me. I can choose to remain happy and calm. Now, does this mean that everyone really has a positive intention with their behaviour? No, it is just a presupposition. Obviously, if you look at individual examples of murderers and despots, then it is hard to find a positive intention behind their behaviours. Hitler, for example, might have thought he had a positive intention with his actions, but it was still what would we would consider "insane".

- **The most important information about a person is *how* that person is behaving.**

  A person's behaviour will give you a great deal of information about their Model of the World and inner screening filters, inner values and beliefs.

- **Everyone is doing the best they can with the resources they have available.**

  This means that we must never judge someone, because how do we know we would not behave in the same way, if we had their lives and walked in their shoes? We always try to do our best with the experience, wisdom and knowledge that we have at the time.

- **There are no un-resourceful people, only un-resourceful states.**
  People have all the resources they need to succeed and to achieve their desired outcomes. When you think like this, you know that everyone can tap into an amazing treasure trove of positive resources, and when they do, they are much more likely to achieve their goals.
- **There is no failure – only feedback (only learning!).**
  Remember the story about Thomas Edison, who was asked, "How did it feel to fail 2,000 times to invent the light bulb?" He replied, "I did not fail. I just learnt how not to do it."
- **Everyone is in charge of their mind and therefore of whatever results from their actions.**
  This means that we all have to take responsibility for how our lives are.
- **The mind and the body are linked.**
  The Unconscious Mind runs the body as well as the emotions, and also remembers everything that has ever happened to you. Your body hears everything you think and say, so when you are being positive, your body will respond to this by feeling energized, uplifted and happy, and when you are being negative your body responds to this by being tired, drained and feeling depressed. As Deepak Chopra says, "Your body is literally eavesdropping on the conversation from your mind."
- **All procedure should increase wholeness and choice.**
  Everything you do should always lead to more health, wholeness and empowerment, so that you have more *choices* available to you as you choose how to be.

Other useful spiritual presuppositions

- **Perception is projection.**
  This means that everything you perceive in your outside reality is the projection of your own inner filters and Model of the World. This is why you only experience reality as you are, never as reality actually is.
- **We either believe that we are the cause or that we are the effect.**
  When we believe we are the cause, we also believe our lives are the way they are because of the way we think, and that there is something we can do to change the situation. When we are the effect, then we

believe our life is the way it is because of other people, our past, the society we live in and so on. We then give our power away and believe there is nothing we can do to change things. This causes us to feel helpless.

Now some people may take this one too literally. If you have neck pain from carrying your daughter on your shoulders it may not be because you feel she is a pain in the neck. It might just be because you wanted to carry her and hear her scream with delight and laughter. So try not to be *too* literal.

However, how you *choose* to perceive the event will be completely your own choice. Let me give you an example. I remember watching a news programme after the Asian Tsunami hit in 2004 and listening to a news reporter on site in Thailand. He was interviewing a man who had just found his little baby boy dead. The news reporter asked the man, "How does it feel to have lost your baby?" The man replied, "I feel grateful, because me, my wife and our other three children have survived, while many others have lost everything." I sat there watching the programme, tears streaming down my face, hugging my own little girls. I felt such awe for this man, who in the face of the worst tragedy that can ever happen to a parent, still managed to find something positive to feel about this terrible event. Everyone would have understood if this man had blamed Life for taking his son away from him, but he chose not to. This did not affect what had happened. What had happened was that his son had died and the only choice he had, in that situation, was how to view this event. Would he view it with fear, blame and negativity? Or would he view it with love? He chose the latter and this choice helped him to be more resourceful on behalf of the surviving members of his family.

Did he cause the Tsunami? Is he somehow to blame for what happened to his son? No. What he did cause was how he chose to perceive the event and that choice defined him as a human being.

- **You either get the result you want or you get excuses.**

Or perhaps you get reasons – perhaps even good reasons. So get rid of the excuses and instead start to work toward manifesting the results your heart feels you are meant to manifest in your life.

Chapter 2
The Workings of the Mind

Your mind is amazingly powerful – the most wonderful computer ever created – and it is truly capable of miracles. Look at everything you have in your life and notice how you have created it from your thoughts. Can you see the incredible creative power behind it? What is the mind, then? What is it made up of? Well, it comprises your Conscious Mind and your Unconscious Mind.

The Conscious Mind

Your Conscious Mind is the logical, thinking, rational part of you, and it is fully formed by the age of five, six or seven. You probably experience it as that internal voice you refer to as "me". The Conscious Mind always asks the question "why" and wants to solve any problems logically. However, if you could logically solve all your problems, you would have done it a long time ago, so we can conclude that our problems are stored within our Unconscious Mind – something I discuss below (see pages 27–8). So the Conscious Mind always tries to find the solution, but it never can, because both problem and solution lie elsewhere – in the Unconscious Mind. The Conscious Mind is very important, but it is fairly limited in what it can accomplish for you on its own. It has been estimated that the Conscious Mind only uses up between 10 and 15 per cent of the brain.

The Conscious Mind has the following qualities, it:
* Holds around 5–9 chunks of information in your awareness at any one time. (A chunk, in NLP terms, is a large bit of information). The rest is screened out by the Unconscious Mind.

- Is sequential, logical, linear
- Asks "Why?"
- Is thinking, awake, analytical, deliberate
- Carries out cognitive learnings
- Seeks the solution
- Is aware of now
- Tries to understand the problem
- Is outcome-oriented

The Unconscious Mind

The Unconscious Mind uses between 85 and 90 per cent of the brain. It processes millions of messages of sensory information every second. The Unconscious Mind is responsible for all your emotions and memories and it also runs your body. You don't have to think about how to make your heart beat, your lungs breathe or your intestines digest food – your Unconscious Mind looks after those things. It runs your behaviours and patterns, often basing them on what it has experienced in the past – *your* past. It is as if it has been programmed to run these particular behaviours. This is why we tend to repeat the same patterns and behaviours as our parents, because our Unconscious Mind was programmed with certain behaviours, or ways of dealing with life, during childhood. And, just like a computer program, every time you run an unconscious behaviour program, it produces the same result. However, as with a computer program, if you make changes, these will produce a different result. Many of your unconscious programs help you to be more effective in life. For example, when you learnt to drive a car, you firstly used your Conscious Mind. You tried to use logic and reason to remember where the pedals were, what they did, how to use the gear stick and what the rules of the road were. But after some time, as you continued practising, you were able to drive the car easily and effortlessly. This is because your Unconscious Mind had taken over, allowing your driving to become more effective and safe. Your car-driving behaviour became unconscious.

The Unconscious Mind has the following qualities, it:

- Is intuitive
- Carries out simultaneous processing
- Is the domain of emotions
- Remembers everything that has ever happened to you and keeps these memories repressed in order to protect you
- Holds resources and provides solutions
- Runs the body
- Is in charge of sleeping, dreaming and altered states
- Is in charge of your whole experience
- Takes everything personally
- Represents all learning, behaviour and change

The Wounded Self and the Wise Inner Self

Sometimes people believe that the Unconscious Mind is all-wise and all-powerful. To explain this I am going to talk about our Wounded Self and our Wise Inner Self – both aspects of the Unconscious Mind (just view these as metaphors rather than being connected with Jungian psychology). The Wounded Self is linked to what I call the "fearful" inner ego – our inner darkness. The Wise Inner Self is linked to our Higher Consciousness – our Higher Self. Our negative inner programming is from the Wounded Self and what heals this is the wisdom communicated to us from the Wise Inner Self. Every time we take steps to heal inner negative programming, we dive deep within our inner darkness, bringing the light from our Wise Inner Self with us, like a divine torch of Higher Consciousness, and we transform the old darkness into light. This causes us to feel lighter, to be lighter and to shine even more brightly.

The Collective Unconscious Mind

The well-known research known as the "100th Monkey Syndrome" gave basis to the idea of the Collective Unconscious Mind. Some scientists had been observing a type of Japanese monkey in the wild for more than 30 years. One day the researchers dropped some sweet potatoes in the sand

and then gave them to the monkeys. One young monkey realized that if she washed the potato it tasted nicer. Within a six-year period all the young monkeys had learnt to wash their potatoes before eating them and had also taught the technique to their parents. Only the older monkeys persisted in eating sandy potatoes. But then, suddenly, all the monkeys started washing their potatoes before eating them. No one knows exactly how this happened, but it is thought that it was after 100 monkeys had learnt to wash their potatoes. Shortly after that other monkeys on nearby islands started washing their potatoes, too, even though they had had no physical contact with the original group. It was as if this new insight had jumped across the ocean, as if somehow the monkeys' minds were linked.

It seemed that the monkeys had a "monkey Collective Unconscious Mind". If this is true for monkeys, then it is not so far-fetched to think that it is also true for humans. Could it be that once a critical number of people possess some information, a certain field is strengthened so that the awareness is picked up by almost everyone? My view is that the Collective Unconscious Mind is a bit like the Internet – you can access information that someone else has put there.

The Collective Unconscious Mind in humans is beautifully illustrated by a story of two American families who both adopted a baby from China. Two years after the adoption, Diana Ramirez wrote about her daughter Mia Hanying's forthcoming birthday on an Internet site for parents who had adopted from the same orphanage. Mrs Funk, who had adopted another little girl named Mia (and who did not know the Ramirez family), saw the posting and began to think. The girls had been found at exactly the same spot after they had been abandoned a week apart, and then taken in, separately and unidentified, by a children's welfare institute. Emails were exchanged and it was noted that the two girls looked very much alike. This was followed by DNA tests, which showed an 85 per cent likelihood that the girls were, in fact, sisters. With unidentified parents this is the highest possible reading. Mrs Funk said in an interview, "It's an awesome thing, a miracle. In the sea of humanity, these kids found each other."

The two families realized that the two Mias were identical twins. Here we have two little souls sharing an immensely strong bond, being separated just a few weeks after birth and ending up on the other side of the world, in separate families, 1,400 miles apart. And by the time they were three years of age their Unconscious Minds had somehow been able to connect with each other through the Collective Unconscious Mind, enabling them to meet up. Amazing! The two girls now talk to each other on the phone regularly and their families meet up as often as they can.

You have probably experienced the Collective Unconscious Mind at work. Has the phone ever rung and you knew who it was before you answered? Or have you ever known something has happened to someone you love, without you having had access to any information about them? Perhaps you think of someone you have not seen for years and then the same day you bump into them, or they give you a call? We are all linked at an unconscious level and the more you love someone, the stronger the link is.

The Conscious Mind, the Unconscious Mind and the Higher Conscious Mind

There is a direct connection between the Unconscious Mind and Conscious Mind, in that they communicate with each other.

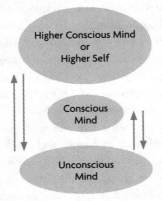

The Conscious Mind may choose to not listen to the communication from the Unconscious Mind, which is what happens when you have a gut feeling that you should take a certain course of action, but then you talk yourself out of it by applying logic and reason. Only later do you realize that you should have listened to your gut feeling all along. For example, this happened to me when I met a man while travelling. My gut feeling told me not to get involved, but my logical mind reasoned that he seemed nice, so convinced me that it was OK to start a relationship. Two years later, with a broken heart, I realized that I should have listened to my gut feeling in the first place – it knew that this relationship would not be good for me. My Higher Conscious Mind (Higher Divine Self) did the best it could and helped me look for all the Positive Learning and insight I needed so that I would not attract this type of relationship to me again.

There is also a direct communication between the Unconscious Mind and the Higher Conscious Mind, and they communicate freely to each other. There is, however, no direct communication between the Conscious Mind and the Higher Conscious Mind, which is why you cannot logically know that the Higher Conscious Mind exists, and also why many who are closely connected to their Conscious Minds rely so heavily on reason and logic and often do not believe in a Higher Conscious Mind. The only way for the Conscious Mind to have an experience of the Higher Conscious Mind is to relax, be still and tune in to the Unconscious Mind, and in that way create a pathway to the Higher Conscious Mind. This is why meditation is so important, because it stills the mind and starts to shut off the internal noise of your brain so that you connect to the inner feeling of peace and happiness, which is already there within you. In this space you can also start to listen to the gentle whispers of your Higher Conscious Mind, which is a very wise aspect of yourself.

Your intuition comes from listening to the messages from your Higher Conscious Mind being communicated to your Conscious Mind via your Unconscious Mind in the form of gut feelings, hunches and sudden insights. We all have these, but the question is, do we listen to them?

> The intuitive mind is a sacred gift and the rational mind is a faithful servant. We have created a society that honours the servant and has forgotten the gift.
>
> Albert Einstein

So honour the gifts within you and apply logic to follow the intuitive guidance you are given.

31

Chapter 3
First-Level Basic Tools and Techniques

We will now start to explore some of the basic tools and techniques of Transformational NLP. We need these before we can move on to the next level. As with any new skill, you first have to learn the basics and once they are cemented in your Unconscious Mind and understanding you can move on to the more advanced levels. These first-level basic tools are suitable for anyone who is new to NLP. If you are already familiar with NLP you can move directly to Chapter 4 (see page 64).

Basic Tool 1: Chain of excellence

This is very simple and merely means that your breathing affects your physiology (posture), and your physiology affects your inner state and feelings, which in turn affect your behaviour. Your behaviour also affects your inner state, which affects your physiology and this affects your breathing. So they are all linked.

One of the quickest ways to change your behaviour and inner state is to change your breathing and physiology. For example, when you are standing up and looking out at the outside world, breathing deeply from your belly, with a smile on your face, you feel positive and resourceful inside. However if you are sitting slumped, looking down, with a sad expression on your face, you will not be able to breathe properly (your diaphragm will be compressed due to your sitting position) and you will feel less energized and resourceful.

Try a quick exercise. Think of something that makes you feel a bit sad and depressed. Notice what posture you adopt. If you are like most people, you will look down, slump and take on a physiology that closes you off from the world.

Now, instead, stand up, with your back straight, look up at the ceiling or sky, with a big smile on your face, and say to yourself, "Yes, yes, yes, yes, yes!" while still trying to hold on to that old thought that made you feel sad and depressed. What happens? That's right! The sad thought disappears because your posture is one of being happy and open, and as your physiology tells your brain, "Hey, I have a happy physiology!" the thoughts that are not in alignment with this happy posture disappear because there is nothing to keep hold of them. Like energy attracts like energy and this means that a happy posture attracts happy thoughts and a sad posture attracts sad thoughts.

How breathing and posture affect our behaviour and vice versa

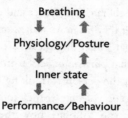

Breathing

Physiology/Posture

Inner state

Performance/Behaviour

Basic Tool 2: Sensory acuity and calibration

Have you had the experience of "just knowing" what your partner is thinking or feeling, without them telling you, or that you "just know" when your child is sickening for something, long before they actually start to develop symptoms? My husband has an uncanny ability of knowing when I am sad or worried long before I have detected it myself, which always amazes me.

So how is this possible? Well, here we are using our natural skills of "calibration" (or "observation" in ordinary language), because it is something that we do all the time; you learn what certain physiologies and expressions mean for certain people. What we are now going to learn is how to do this without performing a "mind read", that is without claiming to know what is in someone else's mind.

Here we will cover techniques on how to use your sensory acuity and calibrate someone else's physiology.

What is sensory acuity?

Your sensory acuity is your ability to use your senses, your vision, your hearing and also your feelings. But why would we want to increase sensory acuity? Remember one of the presuppositions of NLP: one of the most important pieces of information about a person is their behaviour. What they do is more important than what they say. What we are going to look at in sensory acuity are the small changes that take place in a person's physiology, such as in their tone of voice, their breathing, their facial expressions and the slight variations in their posture. Once we are able to notice these changes we can begin to calibrate them and then work out what those changes mean to that person. This is especially important when we want to be able to calibrate the difference between someone's Unconscious Mind's "Yes" and "No" signals, as well as being able to calibrate congruence and incongruence, so that we are able to know whether they mean what they are saying.

We never assume that something means a particular thing until we have calibrated it for that *particular* person in that *particular* context. So when we know that the person is thinking one particular thing we can calibrate the physiology of that. If they then change their thinking to something else, we can calibrate how their physiology changes. Once we have calibrated it, once we see and experience the physiology, then we know what the person is thinking about. We also know when they move from thinking about one thing to thinking about another, because we can calibrate the differences in their physiology. So the whole issue of sensory acuity in NLP is about calibration. Remember: nothing means anything until you have calibrated it, for that particular person and in that particular situation.

What can we calibrate in a person's physiology?

Visual cues

Look at:

- Skin colour – does their skin go from light to dark? Imagine looking at someone in a black-and-white picture. When they are happy they tend to have a "lighter" tone to their natural skin colour, but when they are angry or depressed, they tend to have a "darker" tone. We even have expressions about this in our language: "Her whole face *lit up* with delight" or "His face *darkened* with anger".

- Minute muscle changes. Is their face symmetrical or non-symmetrical? Tense or relaxed?
- Lower lip changes – full or stretched?
- Pupil dilation and whether their eyes are focused or unfocused.
- In which direction do they look – up, down, right, left or in front?
- Breathing – is it rapid or slow? Where is the breathing happening?
- Torso – is their torso tense or relaxed? If it is tense, where do they hold the tension?

Auditory cues

Listen to:
- Volume
- Tone
- Timbre
- Speed
- Pauses
- Rhythm
- Words
- Location of their voice – is it up in the throat or upper chest (higher-pitched, and it can also be a softer voice), or does it come from further down the ribcage (a fuller, deeper voice)?

It is important to know the difference between sensory-based information or a "mind-read". For instance, if you look at someone and think they look sad, then that is a mind-read. If you instead notice that their breathing is shallow and coming from the upper chest, their voice tone is soft and coming from high up in their chest, their eyes look up and to the right and they leave pauses between words, then all of this is sensory based, because it is a description of what you can actually see and hear.

When we are calibrating physiology we want to make sure that we are only ever calibrating sensory-based information. We must switch off our mind-reads, which tell us that we think we know what the other person is thinking and feeling, when in fact we don't.

How to calibrate

Avoid analyzing; you are trying to calibrate with your Conscious Mind. Instead trust your Unconscious Mind. Stay open and attentive at the same time. Go into peripheral vision (expand your awareness to the sides and *behind* you, while still looking at the person. This is in sharp contrast to tunnel vision, when you just focus on what is in front of you). Go inside yourself and imagine taking a step back and taking a snapshot of the other person's physiology in a particular state; say, for example, their physiology when they think of someone they love. Then do the same for their physiology when they think of someone they dislike. Keep doing this until you have built up enough information to be able to calibrate the difference between this person's physiology when they think of someone they love and their physiology when they think of someone they dislike.

How to use sensory acuity in real life

You use your calibration naturally with your friends and family. The better you know someone, the better you know their physiology, as you have built up enough of a data bank, having calibrated their various physiologies in various contexts.

In coaching

In coaching it is essential to be able to calibrate congruence and incongruence in your client as this enables you to find out what is really going on. When a client is "congruent", both the Unconscious Mind and Conscious Mind are in agreement. When a client is "incongruent", the Conscious Mind may want one thing and the Unconscious Mind may want something totally different, so the client is not fully honest about what they are thinking and feeling (the client may not be consciously aware of this, though). You can also tell whether your client is just pretending to give you the right answer or if they are actually telling you their inner truth. Being able to calibrate the client's Unconscious Mind's answer for "Yes" and "No" enables you to calibrate whether what they are saying is congruent with their Unconscious Mind.

Sensory acuity exercises

Find a friend to practise your ability to calibrate correctly by using sensory acuity. If you are pretending to be the client, make sure you do the exercises only when you are in the desired state. For example, start counting (see below) only when you truly feel an inner state of love or a strong state of dislike. In this way you are making it easier for the coach to calibrate the pure state of love or dislike, instead of a mixed state.

Exercise 1. Visual and auditory. Work in pairs. One person takes the role of the client and the other the coach. The client thinks of someone they love: Person A. Think of this person while counting out loud to 10.

Take a break for a few seconds.

Now the client thinks of someone they really dislike: Person B. Think of this person while counting out loud to 10.

Take a break for a few seconds.

Now the client chooses one person at random and lets the coach calibrate which one it is – Person A or Person B. The coach has to get three right in a row. If the coach makes a mistake, start all over again

Exercise 2. Visual. The client thinks of Person A, but this time remains silent. The coach has to use only visual sensory acuity to calibrate.

Take a break for a few seconds.

The client thinks of Person B and is silent. The coach calibrates.

Take a break for a few seconds.

The client now chooses either A or B and the coach has to calibrate which one it is. They have to get three right in a row.

Exercise 3. Auditory. The client thinks of Person A, but this time the coach must not see the client's face, so the client turns their back on the coach. The client counts to 10 while thinking of Person A.

Take a break for a few seconds.

The client thinks of Person B, and again the coach is not allowed to see the client's face. The client counts to 10 while thinking of Person B.

Take a break for a few seconds.

Now the client chooses A or B at random and lets the practitioner calibrate which one it is. The practitioner has to get three right in a row.

Basic Tool 3: Setting up the Unconscious Mind's "Yes" and "No" signals

This is a vital exercise to practise, because as you learn to listen to the wisdom of your own Unconscious Mind you learn how to get your Conscious Mind and Unconscious Mind working together, which allows you to tap into an immense power within. Since your Unconscious Mind consists of between 85 and 90 per cent of your brain capacity and is also linked with your Higher Self, it would be very useful to be able to ask it specific "Yes" and "No" questions.

I have recorded this exercise (an adaptation of the original exercise designed by John Grinder and Carmen Bostic St Clair), so listen to it now, and as you listen to it, be aware of how you feel inside as you answer "Yes" and "No". You can download it at www.nordiclightinstitute.com

Teaching someone to calibrate their "Yes" and "No" signals

Many people are able to learn how to calibrate their own "Yes" and "No" signals. However, some find it very hard. If this sounds like you, then don't worry. Just keep listening to the recorded exercise and you will sooner or later learn how to listen to your Unconscious Mind and trust it. If you are doing this process with someone else, then it is great if they can feel their own "Yes" and "No" signals, but it is also important that you learn to calibrate the difference in the person. *Never tell the person what you calibrate*, as they will start to change their physiology.

I will outline below a simple version for establishing "Yes" and "No" signals in someone else.

For establishing "Yes" and "No" signals in someone else

The following script is for an exercise is for coaches to practise with their clients, as a quick way of being able to read their "Yes" and "No" signals from the Unconscious Mind:

"I am now going to ask you some simple 'Yes' and 'No' questions, so I am able to read your Unconscious Mind's signals for 'Yes' and 'No'. Is that OK?

"Great. So with the following questions I want you to answer 'Yes' and 'No' out loud, and you can have your eyes open or closed, as you wish.

"Are you sitting down? Are you standing up? Are you a woman? Are you a man? Are you in Sweden? Are you in the UK? Are you wearing jeans? Are you wearing a skirt? Do you have brown eyes? Do you have blue eyes? Do you have 15 pink cats at home? Are you standing on your head?" (Keep asking "Yes" and "No" questions until you can calibrate the difference between "Yes" and "No" in your client's physiology. Never tell the client what the difference is.)

Filter to protect against other people's negativity

It is very useful to set up a filter within your Unconscious Mind, to protect you against other people's negativity. This will help you immensely in your life.

Process

Instruct your Unconscious Mind to set up a filter to protect you, so say, "Dear Unconscious Mind, please set up a filter now to protect me from other people's negativity, while still warning me if I am near physical danger. Do you understand?" (Wait to get a "Yes" signal. If you don't, you can also ask it the question: "What is it you need to know and learn so you are able to understand this now?" Wait for the answer, then ask it if it understands. Keep doing this until your Unconscious Mind understands and you get a "Yes" signal.)

"Do you accept responsibility to set up this filter now?" (Wait for a "Yes" signal).

"I now instruct you to set up this filter straightaway, which will protect me from other people's negativity, while still warning me if I am near physical danger." (Wait for your Unconscious Mind to signal with a "Yes" signal when it has done that.)

Basic Tool 4: Building rapport through physiology

Have you ever had the experience of just "clicking" with someone? When you felt as though you had known this person for ages? As you bring that person up in your mind now, what was it about that person that made you instantly click with them? I would guess it was that you had something in common with them. Perhaps you had similar values, were in a similar profession, or came from the same part of the world? Somehow you were like each other. One of the premises of NLP is that when people are like each other they like each other. All this happens at a completely unconscious level.

What is rapport?

The word "rapport" derives from the French word *rapporter* and translates as "to bring back, to return". The English dictionary definition is "a sympathetic relationship or understanding".

So rapport is when we feel a state of trust and understanding. It helps us to feel that we can be open with someone else. Rapport can happen on a one-to-one basis or on a many-to-one basis. Think of the people you have the most rapport with and also how you know that you have rapport with them. Think of how much easier it makes your relationship when you do have rapport with people. Rapport also increases your empathy with others, because it enables you to feel and understand at a deeper level what they are going through.

Rapport also enables you to get on more easily with other people, and you almost certainly have great rapport with your friends (and not such great rapport with the people you don't like so much). The concept of rapport is not new to you, because you have been building it all your life; it's just that you have not been consciously aware of it. Rapport is something we engage in intuitively when we naturally get on with people.

Why build rapport with people?

Having rapport with people enables them to take on board your help and suggestions more easily. This is particularly useful if some of your suggestions might be challenging to them. Say you notice your friend doing something that is not helping her and you would like to offer her some advice. Having great rapport with her as you offer this advice is going to make it much easier for her to listen with an open mind, instead of becoming defensive and angry. Equally, in a job situation, you might have to offer someone constructive criticism. Having rapport with them will make it easier for them to take your advice on board.

As a coach you will have clients coming to you because they have negative inner screening systems, various Problem Strategies and Limiting Beliefs. Now, even if they come to you for help, they often still resist letting some of their problems go and may end up trying to keep holding on to them, employing a variety of techniques: confusion, tiredness, defensiveness, anger, helplessness, pretending to let go but in fact not doing so, boredom, arrogance, insecurity, anxiety, panic and so on. Being in rapport with them, while at the same time "calling their bluff" is vital (you are able to see past their attempts to hold on to the problem). You can see through the smoke screen they put up and, being in rapport with them, you have a much greater chance of pacing and leading them past this smoke screen so you can work on the real problem, which they were trying to hide.

From an NLP point of view it is very important *how* we use our physiology and the way that we say what we say. If you were to imagine a dog: the dog has absolutely no understanding of the words you say (except for a few command words), but will know instinctively how you are feeling. This is because the dog is reading your physiology, your body language, and will also listen to your tone of voice. It is the same with children and adults. Have you ever been with someone who said polite things to you, but you could still *feel* the anger underneath? Or have you ever tried to speak sternly to your child, but been laughing inside, with the result that your child just laughed back and took absolutely no notice of you telling her off? That is because the physiology and the voice tone is far more important in our communication than the actual words. The words are important, too, of course, but when working with rapport, physiology and tone of voice (called "voice tonality" in NLP) are the most important aspects.

Some studies done in the 1970s suggested that our communication was divided into the following: 55 per cent physiology, 38 per cent tone of voice, 7 per cent the words we use. This means that 93 per cent of our communication is unconscious – that is, it is your Unconscious Mind that is communicating, and the Conscious Mind is only using around 7 per cent of the communication style in the form of words. So, for example, if you are really angry with someone, then chances are your

Unconscious Mind will reveal your anger through your body posture and your tone of voice, while your Conscious Mind might still try to be pleasant through your conversation.

How does this work in real life?

If you have to tell your teenager that she has to learn to be more respectful in her communication with you, and you have a physiology of truly loving her, being compassionate with her, and at the same time being full of tough love, because you know she has to learn to be respectful of others, you then say:

"Honey, I want you to speak to me in a way that you would like me to speak to you. It is really important to learn to treat others the way you would like them to treat you. I am your parent, so it is part of my job description to teach this to you. So this means, if you use that way of communicating with me again, there will be consequences. Now I do this because I love you, I want the best for you and I want you to live a happy life. Part of living a happy life means learning how to get on with people."

In this example, both your words and your physiology are showing your child how you would like her to be. If, instead, you were to say the following, while displaying an angry physiology:

"Don't you use that tone with me, Missy! You just wait until your father gets in and I will tell him how rude and impolite you are. You are behaving like such a brat, thinking you rule the universe. Well, let me tell you, while you're living under my roof, you do as I say!"

Your teenager has behaved in the same way, but your response has been different, although you have the same outcome in mind: you want her to learn how to be more respectful and polite. However, which of these two approaches do you think will achieve the better outcome?

If you are talking to someone and you truly know deep within that something works, because it has worked for you, then your physiology and voice tonality (93 per cent) will communicate this to the other person, as well as your words (7 per cent). This will cause the other person to trust you and you will then be able to achieve rapport with them naturally.

Compare this with what happens if you are not sure that something works, because you have not actually experienced it, only read about it. Your physiology will then communicate this state of being unsure (93 per cent) even if with your words you are trying to be sure and confident (7 per cent). This will prevent others from trusting you.

Rapport in coaching

Often I have to say very tough things to my clients, such as with one person I saw, who was depressed, lacked direction in life and allowed others to overrule her, even though she was in her mid-forties. She was otherwise healthy, with a kind heart. Her main problem was that she wanted to avoid arguments at all costs. She had never got on with her mother, who would constantly criticize her and tell her how useless she was. My client had a daughter herself, who did not live with her. Instead she lived with my client's mother, whose home was more than two hours away. This was because the grandmother had decided that my client was unfit as a mother and had literally taken the child away several years ago, without my client having the strength to challenge her. Since she wanted to avoid arguments at all costs, she did not even want to fight for her own child. The problem was, my client and her daughter both wanted to live with each other and neither of them wanted the daughter to live with the grandmother. My client was sitting with me, feeling sorry for herself and blaming the grandmother for all her problems. I knew I had to use very tough love with her to get her to wake up to what was going on, so with great rapport I said:

"Isn't it about time that you grew up? You have a daughter who needs you, so don't you think it is time for you to finally be the mother she needs? Isn't it about time you stopped being so selfish, focusing on avoiding arguments with your mother, instead of focusing on what is best for your own child? Imagine you were a lioness and someone had just taken your cub away. How would you respond?"

My client first looked absolutely shocked. No one had told her that before. But from that moment, she stopped focusing on blaming her mother and instead she dealt with how *she herself* had allowed this situation to happen. Two weeks after her Break-Through coaching session her daughter moved back in with her and however much the grandmother screamed and fought, my client did not back down. She had stepped into her own inner lioness, doing what was best for her cub!

With rapport my challenging words were able to reach my client, because she could feel that I had her best interests at heart. She could feel that I said the words with compassion and love. Compassion, by the way, is not "soft" love. It is a very powerful, tough love, because it acts on spiritual truth. However, there is never any judgment in it and that is why it is so powerful. Imagine if I had said those same words to my client, but with judgment. How do you think she would have responded then? So use rapport with love and compassion.

Formal ways of gaining rapport

These are not the best ones to use as they are done mainly with the Conscious Mind:

Matching is when you match the person's exact movements. For instance they tilt their head to the right, so you tilt your head to the right.

Mirroring is when you become the person's mirror image, so if they cross their legs with the right on top, you cross your legs with the left on top.

Crossover mirroring is when you mirror someone else's physiology without going into the same state. For example, you can mirror someone's breathing by tapping your finger at the same pace as they are breathing in and out. It is useful if the other person is in an emotional state you don't want to be in yourself.

Building rapport through matching and mirroring

1. Posture – the angle of the spine when sitting, the head and shoulder relationship, the upper body and lower body positions
2. Gestures
3. Facial expressions and blinking
4. Breathing – rate and location of the breathing

You have to be very careful when matching and mirroring, because if you are doing it in an obvious way the person you are trying to gain rapport with will feel as though you are mimicking them and that will definitely destroy any rapport!

Building rapport through voice tonality (tone of voice)

1. Voice tonality (tone of voice) – low to high
2. Tempo/speed of speech – slow to fast

3. Quality of tone –distorted to clear
4. Volume of voice – quiet to loud
5. Origin of voice – stomach/chest/throat

Here you just use a similar tone of voice, similar speed and try to generate sound from the same location: stomach, chest or throat. Again, be careful not to come across as mimicking the other person.

Building rapport with words

In order to gain rapport you use similar types of words or you talk about similar experiences and values. This is something you do instinctively and naturally with the people you have the greatest rapport with, as they tend to be the ones you have a lot in common with. So just use your natural rapport-building skills.

More useful ways of gaining rapport

When you stop thinking about yourself and instead fully connect with the compassion in your heart, become *totally present* with the person sitting in front of you, then you will naturally go into rapport. As soon as you start thinking about yourself, then you will go out of rapport.

An additional technique for tuning into the other person's physiology is just to place intention in doing so. This is something I do naturally as a cranial osteopath and I have found it extremely useful. As soon as you tune into the other person you will naturally and immediately go into rapport with them.

You can also tune into their physiology and then lock (hold) that physiology, for example in your neck (with your intention), which then leaves you free to move and talk the way you want. This is called "micro-muscle mirroring" – the tiny muscles in your neck mirror the physiology of the other person.

I have found that practising rapport like this is all I have to do and it feels completely natural. This means that I don't have to think about how to sit, breathe, which words to use and so on, because by tuning into the other person and being fully connected with the compassion inside my heart and being genuinely interested in the other person, I naturally go into rapport unconsciously – instead of using my Conscious Mind to guide me.

Remember how Nepalese people greet one another with "Namaste", which means, "God in me greets God in you". If you have this as your intention, you will easily be able to go into rapport with others.

Pacing and leading

Pacing and leading mean that you first pace the other person in such a way that you gain rapport with them. In order to do this you have to be able to rely on your sensory acuity to calibrate them correctly. You do this by giving the other person your full attention, which enables you to pace what is really going on inside them. This helps you to gain rapport quickly and then you can lead them to follow your guidance, so that you are able to give them advice, or, if you are working with them, take them through various processes and techniques.

When you would like to break rapport

At times it may be necessary to break rapport – perhaps because you haven't got time to talk just now. To break rapport just start to mismatch the other person: break eye contact, move away or change your tone of voice.

Rapport exercises

Exercise 1. Match, mirror and do crossover mirroring of each other's physiology while having a conversation and agreeing on the subject. Or, put in a simpler way, open your heart, be compassionate and place your intent on the other person, so that your physiology is saying, "I like you, I am here for you." Agree also with your words.

Take a break for a few seconds so you change state.

Exercise 2. Now continue having a conversation and agreeing with each other, while mismatching each other's physiology, go out of rapport with the physiology. Here your words are saying, "I agree with you and I like you," but your physiology is saying, "I do not like you, I am not interested in you."

Take a break for a few seconds.

Exercise 3. Now start to match and mirror each other's physiology again, while this time disagreeing with your words. Or, put in a simpler

> way, open your heart, be compassionate and place your intent on the other person, so your physiology is saying, "I like you, I am here for you", but at the same time you are disagreeing with your words.

(Notice what happens in all three exercises. Exercise 3 is the most important exercise for you to master, since it is likely you will have to challenge others with your words and then maintain rapport with your physiology.)

Basic Tool 5: Representational systems

Representational systems are the modalities we use inside our heads to re-present the external world. We represent our thoughts, memories and immediate responses to external stimuli through a continual flow of pictures, sounds, feelings and, to a lesser extent, smells and tastes, too.

The system we use to open mental files is called the "lead system" and it is determined by eye-accessing cues (see Basic Tool 6, pages 55–7). The system we use the most is called the "primary representational system" and it is determined by the predicates (words) a person uses. The more versatile we become at using all systems, the more behavioural flexibility we have and the more enriched our direct experience becomes.

Representational archetypes

Visual

These people tend to stand or sit with their bodies erect, with their eyes up. They breathe from the top of their lungs and talk quickly (describing a series of pictures). They tend to be neat and tidy, because looking good is important to them. They memorize by seeing pictures and are not distracted by noise. They have trouble remembering verbal instructions, but find it easier to remember diagrams and graphs. They are often thin and wiry in body.

Predicates: see, look, view, appear, vision, bright, clear, perspective, show, dawn, reveal, illuminate, visible, foresee, bright, glow, clarify, outlook, imagine, focused, foggy.

Predicate phrases: an eyeful, appears to me, beyond the shadow of a doubt, catch a glimpse of, clear cut, hazy idea, in light of, in view of, mind's eye, paint a picture, crystal clear, seems blurred to me, I can see what you mean, tunnel vision.

Auditory

These individuals breathe from the middle of the chest, often talk to themselves and are easily distracted by noise. They can repeat things back to you easily, learn by listening and usually like talking on the phone. They memorize things by using steps, sequences and procedures. They like to be told how they are getting on and respond to a certain tone of voice or set of words and they want to know what you have to say.

Predicates: hear, listen, sounds, tune in/out, silence, shout, amplify, call, deaf, outspoken, tell, say, melody.

Predicate phrases: blabber-mouth, rings a bell, clear as a bell, clearly expressed, give me your ear, heard voices, hidden messages, hold your tongue, loud and clear, tongue-tied, likes the sound of, tune into this, music to my ears.

Auditory Digital (AD)

These individuals use more Auditory Digital disassociation from their experience to evaluate (i.e. analyze the experience rather than actually feeling it). They are logical and sensible (or at least they think they are). They talk to themselves often and they want things to make sense. They can also have characteristics of the other representational systems.

Predicates: sense, experience, understand, think, process, decide, learn, interpret, analyze, logical, determine.

Predicate phrases: this makes sense to me, I can understand the logic in that, analyze to death, common sense.

Kinaesthetic

These individuals breathe from the bottom of their lungs. They move and talk very slowly. They respond to physical reward and touching and they tend to stand closer to people than a Visual person does. They memorize by doing or walking through something. They want to know if something feels right or they want to test it physically.

Predicates: feel, touch, grasp, get hold of, slip through, catch on, connect with, concrete, solid, soft, tremble, warm, cold, shake, cool, wet, exciting, firm.

Predicate phrases: all washed up, boils down to, come to grips with, get a handle on, get a drift of, hand in hand, hang in there, solid as a rock, take it one step at a time, hold on, hold it, lay cards on table, pain in the neck, pull some strings, slipped my mind, stiff upper lip, it hit home, start from scratch, get in touch with, cool, calm and collected.

Overlapping Representation Systems

This occurs when you take a client from one representational system into another. For example, if you are working with a Kinaesthetic person who has difficulty seeing pictures, you need to take them from Kinaesthetic to Auditory and finally to Visual. You might say, "Remember a time when you were at the beach, *sitting* on the *soft* sand, *feeling* the wind blowing in your face and enjoying the sun's rays *warming your skin*. You can *hear the seagulls, children laughing* and playing, and you sit there *listening to the waves crushing in to the shore*, while *looking out at the horizon, seeing* the crystal-clear blue water and the light-blue sky."

Representational System Preference Test

Assign a number to each of the following statements. Use the following scale to indicate your preferences:

4 = Closest to describing you
3 = Next best to describing you
2 = Next best
1 = Least descriptive of you

1. When I am about to make a decision I do it based on:
   ____ The most logical decision after I have evaluated all the options.
   ____ The decision that looks and appears to be the best.
   ____ The decisions that sounds the best, or that I like the sound of.
   ____ My gut feeling and intuition, or what just feels right.

2. When I am faced with a problem, I find it helps if:
____ I can let my feelings out about what is happening.
____ I can make sense of things in my head.
____ I can talk with someone about it.
____ I can see the bigger picture.

3. I am very:
____ Good at making sense of various data and complex topics, or keeping things ordered and structured.
____ Good at picking up other people's feelings, or feeling intuitively what is going on.
____ Sensitive to the sounds of my environment, or to the tone of voice in others, or to the words they use when they are talking.
____ Influenced by how something looks, or by the appearance of others, or wanting my environment to look nice.

4. When I am stressed I tend to release it by:
____ Moving my body or fidgeting.
____ Watching something, drawing or staring into space.
____ Thinking about it or talking to myself.
____ Talking with a friend or listening to someone.

5. I form an opinion of someone when I first meet them based upon:
____ Their appearance, such as how they dress and look.
____ Their voice tonality (tone of voice) and how they speak.
____ Whether they seem to be sensible and logical.
____ My gut feeling and intuition, or the "vibes" I get from them.

6. When I am thinking of taking a new job I make a decision based upon:
____ Whether the job prospects appear bright and attractive.
____ Whether the job prospects make sense and logic tells me it will be useful.
____ Whether what the job position entails sounds good or if I like the sound of the person I have spoken to about the job.

____ Whether the job feels right for me, or whether my gut feeling and intuition tell me it is right.

7. When I am with other people, I find I most like the people who:
____ Are very lively, talk fast and think fast.
____ Like to stand close to me and talk about feelings.
____ Talk to me a lot and like listening to me.
____ Are very logical, analytical and sensible.

Preference test answers:

Step 1 Copy your answers from the test to here:

1.		3.		5.		7.	
____	AD	____	AD	____	V	____	V
____	V	____	K	____	A	____	K
____	A	____	A	____	AD	____	A
____	K	____	V	____	K	____	AD

2.		4.		6.	
____	K	____	K	____	V
____	AD	____	V	____	AD
____	A	____	AD	____	A
____	V	____	A	____	K

Step 2 Add the number associated with each letter. There are seven entries for each letter.

	V	A	K	AD
1				
2				
3				
4				
5				
6				
7				
Total				

Step 3 The comparison of the total score in each column will give you your relative preference for each of the four major representational systems.

It is a good idea to try to learn to use any of the representational systems for which you received a low score since being able to use all four will help you to communicate in a way that appeals to everyone. This will enable others to get a good feeling about what you are saying to them, so that they can make sense of it, and you will often see this in their faces as they are talking to you.

Additional information for coaches

Coaches and clients

During training and clinical practice sessions, I can very quickly see which representational system a student uses the most while working as a coach and as a client. In order to coach someone, including coaching yourself, it is important to learn how you are as a coach and also as a client. It will make you more efficient and therefore the coaching (of yourself and of others) will be much easier.

Visual

Visual coaches work very rapidly and just want to get on with the exercise, because in their mind they can already see themselves doing it. Their main challenge is when they work with a Kinaesthetic or very Auditory Digital client and they then have to learn *compassion* and *patience* (they can at times become frustrated with a slower client) and learn how to be able to calibrate (observe) their client well.

Visual clients work very rapidly, so you have to make sure you, as the coach, are able to match this. Visual people often describe pictures and metaphors and you might have to ask them what that particular metaphor or picture represents to them. But, above all, you as a coach have to work very, very fast with a Visual client, as they will be able to hide deep, inner problem structures from you and become bored if you are working at a slow pace.

Auditory

Auditory coaches are very sensitive to noise, so they become disturbed by soft music, other people talking, the sound of the chairs scraping on the floor and so on. Apart from that, they usually find it fairly easy to work with most clients, as their pace is somewhere between that of a Visual and a Kinaesthetic person. As a trainer I intentionally position an Auditory person in a place where there is a lot of noise going on and give them an instruction to place their whole awareness on the client and let go of outside distractions. This helps them in their work as a coach later on. I have, on several occasions, worked in clinics where building work has been going on. Of course it is more pleasant when the environment is peaceful, but if there is some noise, then the more relaxed I am about it, the more relaxed my client is going to be. So learning to just accept what is going on is the key to being able to be fully present as a coach.

Auditory clients are usually very easy to work with. They are very sensitive to your voice tonality (tone of voice), how you say the words, as well as all your verbal instructions, so use this. Play with your voice – let it come alive. Use your voice as a tool in facilitating change in your client.

Kinaesthetic

A Kinaesthetic coach often wants to sit very close to the client and may often want to touch them, to show care and attention. Here you have to calibrate (observe) whether your client is happy about this or not. You also have to calibrate whether touching the client is going to help them or not. For example, a client with an attachment to the drama of her emotions may go even deeper into the drama if you touch her sympathetically on her arm, as that may feed the attachment to the drama by giving her attention at the wrong time (see pages 225–6).

A Kinaesthetic coach also has to learn to speed up when working with a Visual client, as they often speak slowly and want to let the client take a long time to process the various steps in an exercise. This will drive a Visual client crazy! Also the client may become bored, as in their mind they have already finished the process a long time before the Kinaesthetic coach tells them the next step.

A Kinaesthetic client is often absolutely fine to work with (it can just take a bit longer, so you may have to try to speed them up a bit) – as long as:

- They do not go into the drama of their emotions.

- They are not a mixture of Kinaesthetic and Auditory Digital. This combination can produce a challenge for the coach. I have noticed the following: the Auditory Digital can block the client from actually *feeling* the feelings, so you have to move past their analyzing brain. The Auditory Digital can also mislead the coach in order to protect the real problem, where very deep emotions are embedded. This can pose problems during the questioning part of a coaching session, but usually once the intervention gets going and you start to access the Kinaesthetic aspect of the client, it becomes easier to work with them. What you have to look out for is the client going into doubt: doubt that the process is working, doubt that they have a real problem, doubt that their emotions are being released – just doubt! Doubt seems to be the alarm bell at which the client's Auditory Digital side comes rushing back in, which then blocks the client again.

Auditory Digital

Auditory Digital students want to analyze an exercise for a long time before doing it, because they want to understand it first and be able to describe logically why you would want to do that specific exercise for that particular problem. I just tell these students to get on with it, and say that we can then analyze the exercise *after* it has been done.

In practice a coach that is very Auditory Digital has to learn to avoid talking too much with their client, so as not to get lost in the talking about the problem instead of detecting its root structure. An Auditory Digital coach also has to learn to trust their gut feelings and allow their inner wisdom to guide them as a coach, rather than trying to rely on logic and reason. They have to learn to let go of doubt and insecurity.

With an Auditory Digital client you have to move past their analyzing, so I gently tap them (physically) on their arm or knee to change their state every time they get stuck in analysis and I often go a bit faster, so that they are unable to grasp what I am doing. I also tell them to stop trying to be in control and that the root cause of their problem lies far deeper than they can reach with logic and reason (if they could have solved their problem by applying logic and reason, they would have solved it a long time ago). And since they are there with me, the problem is obviously still present. Most clients can see the logic in that. This reassures them that they can indeed relax, because that is the wisest choice available, and once that happens the coaching session usually runs very smoothly. I might also choose intervention exercises that are spatial, such as spatial Perceptual Positions (see pages 61–2), to get them to access their Kinaesthetic side and take them out of Auditory Digital, instead of carrying out a Perceptual Position in their head, which in a predominantly Auditory Digital client can get them stuck in Auditory Digital.

Summary

We often possess a mixture of these different types of representational systems and they come to the fore in different contexts. My family would never describe me as being Auditory Digital: I am highly Visual (I speak, think and talk very fast) and I am also Kinaesthetic (I rely on my feelings and intuition and I often stand close to people as I like to *feel* them). However, when I am studying or teaching I am very Visual and Auditory Digital. I am also Auditory, so I like talking and listening to others. As a coach and client I am more on the Visual side, so I work very, very quickly. My challenge as a coach is to develop patience with those who work at a slower pace than mine, and as a client my challenge is to develop acceptance and trust that even if a coach is not working as fast as me I can still benefit tremendously from the exercise.

It is useful to be fluent in all four systems, to give you more options. As a coach it is vital to be able to move between these four systems, so that you are able to pace and lead your client according to the representational system they are using.

Basic Tool 6: Eye patterns

The various eye patterns (see diagram, page 57) are something that NLP is probably most renowned for. However, it is not as simple as thinking that if you ask someone a question and they look up to the right before answering it ("Visually Constructed"), they are lying (because they did not remember the answer, so instead they had to construct it). Again, here we have to use calibration (observation) and you do not know someone's eye patterns until you have calibrated them for that person. John Grinder, one of the co-founders of NLP, said during my Trainer's Training that eye patterns can shift, so that all of them are reversed (from a normally organized person), and also that just one level can shift, so for example the person is normally organized for Visual and Auditory, but Kinaesthetic and Auditory Digital have swapped places. This means that calibration is very important.

Also be aware of synaesthesia. This is when the person is accessing several representational systems simultaneously. For example, someone who is fluent at playing the piano will be able to hear the music while simultaneously moving their hands. They then have an Auditory and Kinaesthetic synaesthesia. If they are reading the notes as well, they have an Auditory, Kinaesthetic and Visual synaesthesia.

Sometimes someone has blocked an area due to a previous traumatic event, such as a man I worked with who could not access his Auditory Digital. I did an eye-movement exercise with him (I drew a big circle in the air with my hand and he had to follow it with his eyes) and spent extra time in the Auditory Digital area, while asking him how old he was the first time he shut this down (stopped being able to access Auditory Digital with his eye movements). He said he was a little boy, so I asked him to imagine that he held this little boy and made him feel safe, and to ask him if he could let him know what had happened. Tears started streaming down his face and it turned out that he had been abused when young and it just did not make sense to him; he just could not understand it. I instructed him to keep on talking to the little boy, silently in his head, and imagine he was like his own little son, and think about what would he say to his little boy. While he did this I was working on his eye patterns, especially in the Auditory Digital region, and within a few minutes he could access that eye movement again.

Questions for eliciting eye patterns

1. "What was the colour of the bedroom you had when you were a child?" "What was the colour of the front door of the house you lived in as a child?" (Visually Remembered)

2. "What would I look like with pink, spiky hair?" "What would your bedroom look like if it were painted orange with purple spots?" (Visually Constructed)

3. "What does Donald Duck's voice sound like?" "What is the tune of the ice-cream van like?" (Auditorily Remembered)

4. "What would I sound like with Donald Duck's voice?" "What would I sound like if I spoke three times as fast?" (Auditorily Constructed)

5. "What was the last thing you said to yourself this morning as you got out of bed?" "What is 34 times 12?" (Auditory Digital)

6. "What does it feel like to walk barefoot on the beach?" "What does it feel like to soak in a warm bath?" "What does it feel like to give someone you love a hug?" (Kinaesthetic)

Eye patterns in a normally organized person
(as you are looking at the client)

VC – Visually Constructed
AC – Auditorily Constructed
K – Kinaesthetic – feeling, senses, touch

VR – Visually Remembered
(seeing what you have seen before)
AR – Auditorily Remembered
(hearing sounds you have heard before)
AD – Auditory Digital (self-talk)

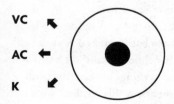
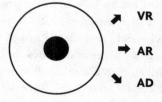

Ask the above questions and make a note of where the client's eyes go as you ask them. As soon as you notice the eye movement, move on to the next question. Also be aware of synesthesia, as the person you are working with may have a strong lead system, which they go to every time to open the mental files (you find the lead system by noticing them going into that eye pattern first every time), before going to the accurate eye pattern.

Basic Tool 7: Perceptual Positions

When I was pregnant with my second child I had a strong feeling that this baby was a girl (I had the same feeling with my first child, although midwives and others told me otherwise). I had been pregnant in between my first and second children, and at that time I was convinced that the baby was a boy, but I miscarried. When I became pregnant this time, it just felt as if the baby was a girl. We had a scan, and were told that it was a boy. I remember just looking at the screen and asking the consultant, "Are you sure? I just have such a strong feeling that this baby is a girl." The consultant smiled and told me to get used to the idea of the baby being a boy, because it certainly looked like that on the scan. That night I had a dream. I dreamed I gave birth to this baby, who was fully clothed. I started taking off the clothes, only to discover a nappy. As I took off the nappy I could see that this baby was, indeed, a little girl.

The next day I did an exercise. I closed my eyes and imagined I could see my baby. What did the baby look like? Oh, she was beautiful. What did I hear from my baby? "Mummy, trust yourself. You know more about me than any scan ever could." What did I feel as I was observing my baby? I felt overwhelming love. What did I perceive about my baby? That she was incredibly wise and strong-willed. What was my highest intention for our relationship? Love. What was the highest intention of that? For my baby to be the person she came here to be.

I then imagined that I floated out of myself and inside my baby. What did I now see as I looked through my baby's eyes back at myself? I saw a mother who wanted the best for her child. What did I hear from this mother? I heard a willingness to listen to things beneath the surface. What did I feel? Love. What did I perceive about this mother? That she loved me and was very wise. What was the baby's highest intention for her relationship with her mother? To grow and experience love. What was the highest intention of that? To grow and develop as a being.

I then imagined that I floated out of my baby, above the two of us. As I now looked down at the relationship, what did I see? I saw two souls sharing an immensely strong love bond. What did I hear? I heard love. What did I feel? Love. What was the highest intention for this relationship? To grow and experience love. What was the highest intention of that? To grow as souls and develop even more in wisdom. What was it that Cissi, down there, needed to know and learn so that she could fulfil her highest intention for her baby? To trust her intuition, trust her Unconscious Mind and trust her own Higher Consciousness, her own Spirit. What did she need to focus on so that she could do that? That all her answers were within her. What advice can you now give to Cissi down there? Just trust herself and her own inner wisdom. Trust the deep connection between her and her baby.

I then floated back inside myself and integrated all these learnings.

From that moment I would often take time to do this exercise and in this way I was able to have a conversation with my baby to check whether she was OK, if she needed anything, what type of birth she would prefer and so on.

So what was it I did? I did Perceptual Positions.

Perceptual Positions

This process increases your perception, awareness and understanding. It changes your filters (that is, how you perceive and interpret through your inner screening system) of the world, and being in Position 2 (see below) gives you a deep unconscious knowledge and insight into another person's filters.

Position 1 – Being inside yourself: seeing, hearing, feeling and perceiving through your own filters.

Position 2 – Being inside the other person: seeing, hearing, feeling and perceiving through someone else's filters. Gives deep unconscious knowledge and insight of the other person's filters.

Position 3 – Being above the two of you, and from a higher level observing the relationship down there. You are here seeing, hearing, feeling and perceiving through filters of being an observer – this increases compassion, detachment and wisdom. This is the position that accesses the wisdom from your Spirit, from your Higher Consciousness.

This exercise is very effective for solving relationship conflicts, as it helps to expand your filters, so that you are able to connect more with your inner compassion and empathy. It also helps you to gain more information, which gives you more choices and enhances your own inner wisdom.

For all the following exercises, imagine that you are your own coach, so you literally read the script to yourself. When I do processes on myself I imagine that I have a little Angel Coach sitting on my shoulder, repeating the script to me, so I follow her instructions. Therefore I will use the word "you" instead of "I".

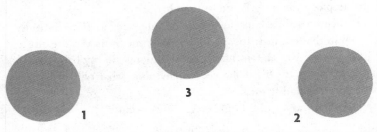

Exercise

Position 1. Close your eyes and imagine that you can see the other person in front of you. Your Angel Coach now asks, "What are you seeing as you look at this other person? What are you hearing from this person? What are you feeling as you are looking at and listening to this person? What are you perceiving about this person? What is your highest intention for your relationship with this person? What is the highest intention of that?" Imagine your Angel Coach keeps asking for the highest intention until you can confirm with the Unconscious Mind signals (see pages 38–9) that this, indeed, is the highest intention. If you are not sure, then at least imagine your Angel Coach asking for the highest intention twice, in order to get to a higher level.

Position 2. Now imagine that you are floating out of yourself and into this other person and you look through this person's eyes back at yourself. Your Angel Coach asks you, "What are you seeing as you look at yourself through this other person's eyes? What are you hearing from yourself? What are you feeling as you are looking at, and listening to, yourself? What are you now perceiving about yourself when you look through this person's eyes? What is this person's highest intention for your relationship? What is the highest intention of that?"

Position 3. Now float out of this person to a position high above the two of you, so you are in a position of being a Wise Observer. Your Angel Coach now asks you, "What are you now seeing as you are observing these two people down there and their relationship? What are you now hearing from them? What are you feeling as you are observing them down there? What are you now perceiving about this relationship? What is the highest intention for this relationship? What is the highest intention of that? What is it that you, down there, need to know and learn so you are able to fulfil your highest intention? What do you need to focus on so you are able to do this? What do you need to know and learn so that you can do this? What advice can you give to yourself so that you are able to do this? Is this in alignment for the highest good of all concerned?"

Then float back inside yourself and integrate all your learnings. Now imagine that you move out into the future and see, feel and notice how you are being now, enriched with all your insights and learnings. Then come back to now.

You can also do this exercise spatially. Find three positions on the floor, which represent Positions 1, 2 and 3 and carry out exactly the same exercise.

Start by being inside yourself in Position 1, looking at this other person being imagined standing in Position 2. Imagine your Angel Coach asking you, "What are you now seeing as you are looking at this other person?" And then they ask all the other questions for Position 1.

Then instead of imagining you are floating outside yourself and inside the other person, you just walk to the Position 2 spot on the floor and now imagine you are inside this other person looking back at yourself (and then look at Position 1 on the floor). Your Angel Coach now asks you, "What are you now seeing as you are looking at yourself through the eyes of this person?" And then she asks all the other questions for Position 2.

Then you do the same with Position 3. So you walk to Position 3 and here your Angel Coach says, "Now when you are in this position of being a Wise Observer, looking at yourself over there (pointing to Position 1) and this other person over there (pointing to Position 2), what are you now seeing?" And then your Angel Coach asks all the questions for Position 3.

Then you walk back to Position 1 and integrate all your learnings and insights. After that you imagine you have a future timeline in front of you and you start to walk out into the future (so walk out onto this imaginary future timeline) integrating all your learnings and insights into your future.

Perceptual Positions with money

You can also do this exercise with energies in your life, such as money. When I took a client through the following exercise, enabling her to heal her relationship with money, she received a large cheque from an unexpected source just a few months later and several work opportunities came her way. Another client worked on her relationship with money and being able to earn money through her creative writing (we did a Break-Through Process, and one of the exercises involved Perceptual Positions in relation to money) and only a few weeks later she had a movie manuscript accepted by a national television company and a hefty cheque for the first advance payment.

Exercise

Position 1. Close your eyes and imagine that you can see the energy of money in front of you. Your Angel Coach now asks you, "What are you seeing as you are looking at the energy of money in your life? What are you hearing from money? What are you feeling as you are looking at and listening to money? What are you perceiving about money? What is the highest intention for your relationship with money? What is the highest intention of that?"

Position 2. Now imagine yourself floating out of yourself and into the energy of money, and looking through the energy of money back at yourself. Your Angel Coach now asks you, "What is money seeing, as money is looking at you? What is money hearing from you? What is money feeling as money is looking and listening to you? What is money perceiving about you? What is money's highest intention for your relationship? What is the highest intention of that?"

Position 3. Now float out of the energy of money and to a position high above the two of you, so that you are in a position of being a Wise Observer. What are you now seeing as you are observing the relationship down there between you and money? What are you now hearing from this relationship? What are you feeling as you are observing this relationship? What are you now perceiving about this relationship? What is the highest intention for this relationship? What is the highest intention of that? What is it that you, down there, need to know and learn so you are able to fulfil your highest intention for your relationship with money? What do you need to focus on so you are able to do this? What do you need to know and learn so that you can do this? What advice can you give to yourself so that you are able to do this? Is this in alignment for the highest good of all concerned?

Then float back inside yourself and integrate all your learnings.

Now imagine you move out into the future and see, feel and notice how you are being now, enriched with all your insights and learnings. Then come back to now.

Chapter 4
Neuro Programming

Submodalities

Many years ago I was trekking in Nepal. I was really fit at that time, being 22 years of age and having just won a kung fu competition. As my friend and I started trekking we realized that this was really hard work. I thought before I started out that you just go up one mountain and that was it. I didn't realize that you went up one mountain, and then walked down it, only to go up another mountain, then down that one, up the next one, and so on. One day we were trekking uphill for eight hours. It was exhausting. Several times we just fell down laughing because we were so tired. As we were taking one step at a time, hands on thighs to help us up, we saw a Nepalese man speed up with a huge pack on his back. He was just skipping up the mountain. Another such man took pity on us and put his hands on our backpacks and literally pushed us up. It was rhododendron season, so blossoms were everywhere; they were stunning. The scenery was amazing, fresh and untouched. After eight long hours we reached our destination for the day and as we stepped into a little guesthouse in a tiny village perched on the mountain, we could smell food cooking and hear the welcoming sound of a crackling open fire and the light chatter of other trekkers. Brilliant, we thought, there are others here, too. After a long day trekking it was always nice to talk to other people in the evening. As I went up to the fire I had a shock. The trekkers sitting there were two older women in their seventies. As I saw them, my jaw dropped, and I asked them, "How did you get up here? Did you fly?"

They just laughed and said, "No. We came the same way you did."

I shook my head in disbelief and could see that they were not particularly fit. One had arthritic knees. How did they do it? Here I was, fit and young, and they were over 50 years older than me, but they had come up the mountain the same way as we had.

It turned out that their grandchildren had been trekking and had sent them a postcard from Kathmandu, and they had thought, "We'd like to do that too!" So they booked flights to Nepal. They didn't go on an organized trip, but arranged everything themselves and the only help they had was from a Nepalese guide, who showed them the way.

Later on, as we were sitting chatting, I turned to one of the women and asked her, "What's your secret? How did you do it? I know how hard this trek is, so how have you managed to do it?"

She leaned closer and whispered in my ear, "Honey, you just picture it in your mind, and you know deep inside your heart that you can do anything – *anything* – if you just put your mind to it."

The next morning we got up very early and started putting on our cold, salty, stiff clothes and then set off. It was a fine day and we walked downhill for several hours into a beautiful valley to a village famous for its hot springs. Later that evening we were lying in these springs when some other trekkers told us about another trek, which was supposed to be amazingly scenic. The only problem was, if we wanted to do this trek instead, we would have to climb the same mountain we had just come down, to the same village where we had met the two women, and from there head in a different direction. We thought about it for a second and then said to each other, "Let's do it!"

The next morning, we again got up early, put on our cold, even stiffer clothes, and embarked on the long climb up this monster of a mountain. After a while I started to think, "This is just too hard. Why am I finding this hard? I should be really fit! How can this be harder than doing full-contact kung fu?" And as I was thinking those thoughts I had a dark picture inside of me, drained of all vitality. Then I remembered the wise woman's words, "Just picture it in your mind and know deep in your heart that you can do anything – *anything* – if you just put your mind to it."

And that is exactly what I did and instead of that old dark, drained picture, I imagined myself skipping up the mountain, like the Nepalese man, singing and laughing, being full of beans. I made the picture bright and sunny, with glowing colours of yellow and orange, full of vitality. Somehow I now seemed to fly up this mountain. Although the trek still took around eight hours, it seemed like eight *easy* hours.

I knew that this woman had given me a great gift – the gift to use my mind to help me to achieve my goals, even when that goal involved a tough mountain to climb.

This was before I had started to learn about NLP and what this woman taught me was to work with programming the way I used my brain, by using my submodalities.

Using submodalities

Submodalities are the "finer distinctions" within the modalities. The modalities are: the Visual, the Auditory, the Kinaesthetic, the Gustatory and the Olfactory. For instance, within the Visual modality the finer distinctions are, for example, if the picture you are creating inside your mind is in black and white or colour, if it is near or far, if it is framed or panoramic, what the size of the picture is, whether it is a movie or a still, and so on. Here is a list of various submodalities within the modalities of Visual, Auditory and Kinaesthetic:

	What you say to yourself or to the other person	
Visual submodalities	When you think of X [whatever the client is working on], do you have a picture?	
Colour	Is the picture in black and white or colour?	
Scale	Is it near or far?	
Brightness	Is it bright or dim?	
Location	Where is it located? (Up, down, right, left, in front?)	
Disassociation/ association	Can you see yourself in the picture (disassociated) or are you looking through your own eyes (associated)?	

Size	What is the size of the picture?	
Number	Is it just one picture or a number of pictures?	
Focused/unfocused	Is the picture in focus or out of focus?	
Focus: changing or steady	If it is focused, is the focus changing or steady?	
Framing	Is the picture framed or panoramic?	
Movie or still	Is it a movie or a still?	
Auditory submodalities	Are there any sounds in the picture? If so, what type of sounds?	[If there are no sounds, move straight down to Kinaesthetic.]
Location	Where is it located?	
Direction	Which direction does it come from?	
Internal/external	Is it internal or external?	
Volume	Is it loud or soft?	
Tempo	Is it fast or slow?	
Pitch	Is it high-pitched or low-pitched?	
Pauses	Are there any pauses in the sound, or is it constant?	
Kinaesthetic submodalities	Are there any feelings in the picture? What type of feelings? Where is that feeling located (inside or outside your body)?	If the feeling had a colour, what would it be? Which direction does this feeling move in?

Size	How big is the feeling?	
Shape	Does it have a shape or a form?	
Intensity	How intense is the feeling?	
Still/moving	Is it steady or moving?	
Pressure	Is there any pressure?	
Temperature	Is it hot or cold?	
Weight	Is there any weight to the feeling?	

In NLP we are more interested in the context, structure and process of the Internal Representation than the content. The Internal Representation is how you internally represent something to yourself, and when you find out the submodalities of that Internal Representation you get all the tiny details of that internal picture.

If you change the structure of the Internal Representation, that is you change the submodalities of the Internal Representation, the meaning of that representation changes.

What do the submodalities do for us?

The submodalities give meaning to our Internal Representation. For example, if I were to ask you to picture a beautiful beach, you would be able to do that, and the content of that picture would be fairly similar to other people's. But the picture would have different meaning to different people, depending on the submodalities you stored the picture in. Some people would say, "I love beaches." Others would say, "I hate beaches!" Others would say, "I like beaches, but I hate the sun." The content is the same, but the submodalities the picture is stored in determine what the picture means to different people.

Our submodalities give meaning to our Internal Representations.

Why would we want to discover submodalities and learn how to change them?

If you think about the submodalities being like the programming language your brain uses, then when you learn *how* to use this inner-brain programming, you learn how to run your own neurology. This means you have more *choices* available to determine how you choose to be.

When you change your submodalities you change the *meaning* of your Internal Representation, which also changes how you feel. So the way we feel about an Internal Representation is because of the meaning and the submodalities. This directly affects the *behaviour* that results from a particular Internal Representation, because of the meaning and the submodalities it is stored in. When we learn to discover what the submodalities of an Internal Representation are, then learn how to change them, we can change the meaning of this particular Internal Representation, which changes the way we feel about it, which then also changes the behaviour that it generates.

Finding the driver

A "driver" is the particular submodality that, when it changes, causes all the others to change with it. When you change the driver, it will have a great impact. You can only discover the driver by calibrating yourself or the person you are doing the exercise with, when you do contrasting analysis (this is when you compare the submodalities for two separate Internal Representations, so you are able to notice the ones that are different). You confirm this when you do "Mapping Across" (here you map across the submodalities you found were different when doing contrasting analysis – see the exercise on pages 73–8). *The driver is the difference that makes the difference.* Common visual drivers are location, association and disassociation.

Think of someone you accept whole-heartedly. Just picture this person in your mind and notice where that picture is located in your mind's inner screen. Is it up or down, to the left or right, or directly in front of you? Then "clear the screen" and think of someone you often criticize; someone you tend to judge and disapprove of. Notice where that picture is located. Is it up or down, left or right? Or is it directly in front of you? Are the two locations different? I guess they are. Now move the picture of the person you criticize to the location of the person you accept. Notice whether that makes you feel differently about the person. Some people just refuse to do this exercise because their Unconscious Minds are not happy about them accepting this person.

Other drivers are "association" and "disassociation". When you are associated you are *in* the picture, inside your body, looking through your own eyes. When you are disassociated you step out of your body, so that you can see yourself in the picture as if you were looking at a photograph of yourself.

I have noticed that you can also have a driver in the other modalities, such as, for example, the feelings in the picture (it's quite common for the colours of the feelings to be a driver), or the sounds in the picture (less common). The only way for you to find out your driver, or another person's, is to use your calibration skills (see pages 33–7).

Eliciting submodalities

When you carry out a submodality technique you need to have your submodality checklist and a pen handy so that you can make a note of them quickly.

A few key points to note when you are eliciting submodalities:

- Speed – do it quickly. For most of us it is hard to hold a picture in the mind for a long time, so by asking the questions quickly this makes things easier. Also we want to catch the submodality as it is now, rather than changing it. If you elicit the submodalities too slowly, by speaking too slowly, such as, "Is the picture in black and white [pause] or colour?" you can end up with first trying the picture out in black and white and then in colour. So avoid this by saying the questions really quickly. You also do not want to give yourself, or the person you are working with, any time to think.
- You first elicit visual submodalities, then you ask, "Are there any sounds in the picture?" If "No", skip this bit. It is fairly common for pictures not to have any sounds. If "Yes", you then ask what type of sound? And then you go through all the auditory submodalities. Then you ask, "Are there any feelings in the picture?" If there aren't,

skip this bit. However, I have actually never experienced a client who had no feelings in connection to an Internal Representation.

When you are experienced with eliciting submodalites, or if you are working in a setting when you just cannot have access to a submodality checklist, you can bring in submodalities in informal or spontaneous ways.

As I am an osteopath, I use submodalities with my patients in a more informal way. During treatment I cannot use pen and paper, as that would prevent me from performing the osteopathy, so I have to rely on my memory. For example, I list the submodalities of them being in pain and when they are feeling healthy and happy. Then I change their submodalities from pain to the submodalities they have when they are happy and healthy.

Submodalities can also can come up as a spontaneous occurrence. One of my NLP students, a nurse, phoned me just a week before the NLP training was due to start. Weeks earlier she had dislocated her hip, leaving her feeling panicky and anxious. She was crying on the phone, feeling bad just talking about it. She also happened to mention that she did not understand submodalities. Great, I thought, let's do a Mapping Across exercise.

I quickly asked her if she could remember when she dislocated her hip. Of course, she said; it was all she could think about. Great, I told her, so when you think about that, do you have a picture? Yes, she did. OK, so is that picture in black and white or colour? Near or far? Framed or panoramic? What is the size of the picture? Where is the picture located? Is it a movie or a still? Are you in the picture so you can see your own body in it (disassociated) or are you looking through your own eyes (associated)? Are there any sounds in the picture? What types of sounds? Where are they? Loud or soft? Internal or external? Any feelings? What type of feelings? Where are they? What is the movement of the feelings? Size? Shape? Colour? Weight? Pressure?

Now clear the screen of that information. How would you have liked to have handled the situation instead? As you think about that, do you have a picture? Is that picture in black and white or colour? Near or far? Framed or panoramic? What is the size of the picture? Where is the picture located? Is it a movie or a still? Are you in the picture so you can see your own body in it (disassociated) or are you looking through your own eyes (associated)? Are there any sounds in the picture? What type of sounds? Where are they? Loud or soft? Internal or external? Any feelings? What type of feelings? Where are they? What is the movement of the feelings? Size? Shape? Colour? Weight? Pressure? Now clear the screen from that and bring up that first old picture.

I then changed her original submodalities to the submodalities she had in the picture of how she wanted to have handled the situation instead. This took only a few minutes. Afterwards she was really calm, and she said, "I have no idea what you did, but I feel great now."

When do you use submodalities?

We use submodalities when we do Mapping Across.

NB: Use Mapping Across only for minor unwanted states and behaviours that are highly contextualized.

Mapping Across

Here we elicit the submodalities of two Internal Representations, one of a desired state and one of a non-desired state. Then we change the submodalities of the undesired state into the submodalities of the desired state. We can use this for changing states such as unmotivated to motivated, confused to understanding, judgmental to accepting. It is also very useful to change a food you really like into a food you do not like, or the other way around. What you have to remember is to use it within the same logical type, so, for example, food with food, drink with drink. When I was pregnant and wanted to stop drinking coffee, my coach elicited the submodalities of coffee and then mapped that across to the submodalities elicited when I was imagining drinking liquidized salted, fried herring. It worked. I then could not drink coffee or eat tiramisu or even coffee-flavoured ice cream, until I one day decided to change the submodality of coffee back when my baby girl was a year old.

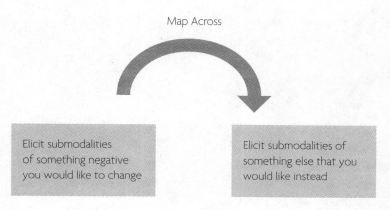

Map Across

| Elicit submodalities of something negative you would like to change | Elicit submodalities of something else that you would like instead |

Here is an example of mapping across in practice, when you have to improvise because the client has difficulty accessing visuals.

Negative state
Not enough money to be able to provide for myself and my family

When you think of that (not having enough money to be able to provide for yourself and your family), do you have a picture?	Initially my client did not have a picture – only feelings, so we had to do overlapping submodalities, starting with feelings, then Auditory, then Visual. Even so, she did not get much that was visual, just blackness.
Is the picture in black and white or colour?	Black.
Is it near or far?	It is both – it is all-over blackness.
Bright or dim?	Dark.
Where is it located?	All over my visual field.
What is the size of the picture?	No size – just big blackness.
Can you see yourself in the picture (disassociated) or are you looking through your own eyes (associated)?	Through my own eyes.
Is the picture focused or unfocused?	It is just black.

If the picture is focused, is the focus changing or steady?	Steady.
Is the picture framed or panoramic?	Panoramic.
Is it a movie or a still?	A still.
If it is a movie, is it fast, normal or still?	
Is it just one picture or a number of pictures?	
Are there any sounds in the picture?	[If there are no sounds, move straight down to Kinaesthetic.] No sounds.
Where is it located?	
Which direction does it come from?	
Is it internal or external?	
Loud or soft?	
Fast or slow?	
High-pitched or low-pitched?	
Are there any pauses in the sound, or is it constant?	
Are there any feelings in the picture? What type of feelings? Where is that feeling located (inside them or outside them)? If the feeling had a colour, what would it be? Which direction does this feeling move in?	Sad and empty. Inside my gut. Black and heavy. A heavy pressure pushing in on me.
What is the size of the feeling?	Big.
Does it have a shape or a form?	Round.
What is the intensity of the feeling?	Intense.
Is that steady or moving?	Steady.

Any pressure?	Enormous pressure.
Is it hot or cold?	
Any weight to the feeling?	Really, really unbearably heavy.

Outcome state
Being able to earn enough money to provide for myself and my family

When you think of your state (being able to earn enough money to provide for myself and my family), do you have a picture?	Again, initially my client said "No". She could just feel feelings, so we did overlapping submodalities here too, meaning we started eliciting submodalities first in Kinaesthetic, then in Auditory and lastly in Visual.
Great! Is the picture in black and white or colour?	Full colour – vibrant happy colours.
Is it near or far?	Near.
Bright or dim?	Bright.
Where is it located? (Up, down, right, left?)	In front.
What is the size of the picture?	Big.
Can you see yourself in the picture (disassociated) or are you looking through your own eyes (associated)?	Body is in it (associated).
Is the picture focused or unfocused?	Focused.
If focused, is the focus changing or steady?	Steady.
Is the picture framed or panoramic?	Panoramic.
Is it a movie or a still?	A movie.
If a movie, is it fast, normal or still?	Normal.
Is it just one picture or a number of pictures?	
Are there any sounds in the picture? If so, what type of sounds?	[If no sounds, move straight down to Kinaesthetic.] Birds singing.

Where is it located?	All around and yet inside me.
Which direction does it come from?	
Is it internal or external?	Internal and external.
Loud or soft?	Pleasant.
Fast or slow?	Moderate.
High-pitched or low-pitched?	Medium.
Are there any pauses in the sound, or is it constant?	Just like birds singing.
Are there any feelings in the picture? What type of feelings?	Happy, light, full feeling. A feeling of being satisfied, similar to after a nice meal.
Where is that feeling located (inside or outside them)?	In my gut and chest.
If the feeling had a colour, what would it be?	Golden, yellow and orange colours, sunny colours.
Which direction does this feeling move in?	Radiates out from my chest, like a shining star in my heart.
What is the size of the feeling?	Big.
Does it have a shape or a form?	Circular, globe-like.
What is the intensity of the feeling?	Happy and calm.
Is that steady or moving?	
Any pressure?	
Is it hot or cold?	Comfortably warm.
Any weight to the feeling?	Light.

Because my client was so Kinaesthetic and could not initially access Visual and only feel the feelings, we had to start with Kinaesthetic and then move up to Auditory and then finally do Visual. For the Mapping Across, I then also started from Kinaesthetic. I first looked at the submodalities for each state and noticed which ones were different (contrasting analysis) and then I mapped it across by doing the following:

I read this out to my client:

"So now think about not being able to provide for yourself and your family. You know that old, sad and empty feeling in your gut, which is black and heavy; a heavy pressure pushing in on you? Change that now so that it becomes a happy, light, full feeling of being satisfied, similar to after you've had a nice meal. And now drain away everything that is old, black and heavy and instead make the colours golden, yellow and orange; all those sunny colours [changing the colours was my client's driver – she especially changed her physiology when sunny colours came and spread to her chest], and now let that happy, light feeling and all those colours of golden, yellow and orange start to radiate out from your chest, like a shining star in your heart. And let that spread now from your heart and chest to your gut and intensify that even more, making your whole gut and chest fill with happy, light, satisfied feelings, and full of yellow, gold and orange sunny colours. And it feels comfortably warm and light.

And now bring in birds singing so that you can hear them singing all around you and yet inside of you. It is a pleasant sound.

Now drain away that old blackness and instead turn the picture into full colour – vibrant happy colours. Let that picture be near you, bright, and move it so it is in front of you. Make it big. See yourself in the picture and make that picture focused and the focus steady. Make the picture panoramic and make it into a movie, with normal speed."

Now because my client had had problems being able to visualize, and also because she kept saying that everything just seemed black and heavy and she could not see a way out, I got her to explore various ways in which she could earn money so that she could provide for herself and her family. She chose four specific areas. Then we looked at one area at a time and I asked her to picture each area. We then changed the submodalities of that picture so that it had the same submodalities as her desired outcome picture. This helped her Unconscious Mind to see more clearly the different ways it had available to it to be able to provide for herself and her family, and this gave her more options.

How to play with the exercise to gain more spiritual wisdom

I then also got her to float up to a sacred mountain top and sit there, so high that she could clearly see her life down here. I then asked her to invite her Wise Higher Self and ask it what the Positive Learnings were for her, so that she could heal this fully now? What was it her Wise Higher Self wanted her to know and learn so that she could move forward in her life, being able to provide for herself and her family? What was it her Wise Higher Self wanted her to pay attention to so that she could do that?

What was the result of this exercise? One year later my client had tripled her income!

What would you normally do?

Usually you would start with all the Visual submodalities, moving on to the Auditory and finally on to the Kinaesthetic. But we are all unique, so you just have to be open, intuitive and willing to play with the situation. With this particular client, the only submodalities she could get were Kinaesthetic. If I had forced her to find Visual, I would have been pushing her and probably become tense myself; we would not have been able to continue. But I knew she would not be able to do it, and that this was just her own inner block that we had to move around. She was literally drowning in her own negative feelings and could just not see a way out. So helping her move through that helped her Unconscious Mind enormously.

Mapping Across for self-healing

Imagine your Angel Coach (see page 61) saying to you,

"Now think of something you would like to change. As you think of that, do you have a picture?"

Now elicit the submodalities of that picture. Go through the questions on the submodality checklist (see pages 66–8) and write down your answers *quickly*.

Your Angel Coach says, "Now think of what you would like to have, be or do instead. When you think of that, do you have a picture?"

Then elicit the submodalities of that picture and write down the answers *quickly*.

Now look at the two lists of submodalities and notice the difference. Then either ask someone to map the submodalities for you (do Mapping Across as I did with my client on pages 73–8). This is easy if they are trained in NLP. If the person is not trained in NLP, then write it out for them like a script that they can read out to you.

Then your Angel Coach says, "Imagine floating up to a sacred mountain top and sit up here, so high that you can clearly see your life down there. Now invite your Wise Higher Self to sit up here with you and ask them what the Positive Learnings are for you, so you can heal this fully now. What does your Wise Higher Self want you to know and learn so you can move forward in your life? What does your Wise Higher Self want you to pay attention to so that you can do that? What do you need to focus on? Then float back down from this mountain, into your life and integrate all your new learnings and insights."

This is a very useful exercise to do on your own and also with others. If you want to, you and a friend can read this exercise out loud. There is also a similar exercise recorded on the download accompanying this book at www.nordiclightinstitute.com

Change negative feelings into positive feelings

Let those positive feelings enrich your life – past, present and future:

1. Think about someone or a situation that makes you feel angry, irritable, negative, worried or anxious. What happens just before you experience these feelings? Is it the way someone looks at you, what someone says or something you see, hear or even think? Notice what it is that triggers these inner feelings. Notice which negative feelings you experience and where in the body they occur. If these negative feelings had a colour, what colour would they be? Which direction do they move in?
2. Open your eyes and shake off this feeling.
3. Think now about a time when you felt truly wonderful: a time when you were filled with happiness, energy, enthusiasm, love and other positive feelings; a time when you were bubbling inside with Life Energy, hope and curiosity, or any other positive feelings you think would be good for you.

4. Where in your body do you feel these feelings? Which colours are they? Which direction do they move in? Do they move backward, forward, clockwise, counter-clockwise, up or down? Most feelings spin in a certain direction, so notice which direction they spin in.

5. Now let your positive feelings start to spin faster and faster and let the colours become more and more intense. Let these positive feelings and colours spin so fast that they start to fill your whole body, and feel, see and notice how these feelings fill all of you, and how they wash away those previous negative feelings and colours until you are completely filled with pure positive feelings and colours. Now let these positive colours and feelings expand even more, so that they start to fill the area around you, too.

6. Now float above, high into the sky, to a beautiful sacred mountain top. And from here you can see your whole life down there as a Timeline. Notice where your past is and where your future is. Also note whether there are any areas on your Timeline that look dark, grey, foggy or cold.

7. Now let all your positive feelings of _____ [state specific feelings] start to spin even faster and imagine how you hold a sacred hosepipe in your hands. Feel, see and notice how these positive colours of _____ [state specific colours] start to flow into this hosepipe and now turn the hosepipe toward your past and let these positive colours of _____ [state specific colours] flow inside your past, filling your whole past with wonderful positive colours, so that your whole past becomes filled with positivity and good feelings, until your whole past Timeline shines and sparkles with the colours of _____ [state specific colours]. These positive colours of _____ [state specific colours] exist within you in abundance and the faster you let them spin inside you, the more of them you create. When your whole past Timeline is filled with these beautiful colours, turn the hosepipe toward your future Timeline and fill your future with the colours of _____ [state specific colours], until your whole future shines and radiates with _____ [state specifics]. Then turn the hosepipe toward the now and fill your present moment with _____ [state specifics], and feel, see

and notice how these colours of _____ [state specific colours] float inside you right now, inside every cell of your body, and fill your whole mind. Feel, see and notice how you breathe in these amazing positive colours of _____ [state specific colours], just as you are sitting here now, breathing in and out. Continue breathing in and out these colours, filling you up with _____ [state specific colours].

8. Now invite your Wise Higher Self to be up here with you on this sacred mountain top. Ask your Wise Higher Self what the Positive Learnings are for you, so that you can fully heal? What do you need to pay attention to so you can heal this? Then thank your Wise Higher Self and float back inside the now and integrate all these positive feelings, colours, insights and learnings deep inside you.

9. Now move out into the future, to next week, and feel, see and notice how you are different now that you are filled with _____ [state specific feelings and colours previously stated]. See yourself a month from now filled with _____ [state specific colours and feelings previously stated], in six months time, in a year and notice how different you are. Also take time now to imagine being in a situation that in the past would have caused you to go into those old negative feelings, and now instead you feel, see and notice yourself dealing with it so differently, enriched with all your positive colours and feelings. See and feel how you flood these situations with all your positive colours and feelings of _____ [state specific feelings and colours stated]. So go now into the future and continue to be filled with _____ [state specific colours and feelings stated], and let these colours and feelings expand and grow all the way out into the future, and keep doing this now all the way into eternity. And there in eternity you meet your most evolved Spiritual Self, who takes you into a Chamber of Treasures. You walk inside and there your Spiritual Self gives you a gift, which will help you on your journey through life. Notice what this gift is, and what it represents to you. Thank your Spiritual Self and then bring this gift with you and let its essence float inside every day for the rest of your life, all the way from eternity back to now.

10. Then, when you are in the now, take a moment to reflect upon everything you have in your life that you are grateful for, and once you have done that, and are ready to live your life to the full, enriched with all your positive insights and resources, then and only then can you open your eyes.

This exercise enables you to change the way in which your brain reacts to a certain situation or a specific person, so instead of going into a negative reaction, you are able to choose to be different, by being filled with positive feelings and resourcefulness. This gives you more options, and therefore more freedom – freedom to choose to be the person you want to be. It also helps you to connect more with your Divine Source of spiritual wisdom, abundance and happiness, which exists within you.

The wisdom of a five-year-old

I did the exercise above with my younger daughter, Natasha, when she was only five years old, albeit as a simplified version. She felt very angry and was building up to a tantrum. I asked her if she wanted me to help her feel happy again and she said, "Yes". I then asked her where she was experiencing the feelings and she said she had them inside her head. They were black, grey and brown. She experienced these feelings as a monster living inside her, which she called "Monstris".

I asked her to think about when she felt happy, filled with energy and love and where in the body she felt these feelings then. She pointed to her heart and stomach and said those feelings were yellow, white, pink, light blue and turquoise. I asked her to let those happy feelings start to spin faster and faster inside her; so fast that they would start to fill her whole body, all the way up to her head and then let them continue to spin faster and faster until those old colours of black, grey and brown had disappeared, a bit like when you put dirty clothes into the washing machine and it just keeps spinning until the whole wash is clean. Natasha was sitting on the floor, cross-legged, eyes closed and moving her head in ever-faster circles as she imagined these positive colours spinning faster and faster inside herself. She looked so cute! Suddenly she looked up and asked, "Mummy, can we put Monstris in the washing machine, just as we put Teddy in there when he is dirty?" I replied that this was a fantastic idea. She laughed and laughed, with her eyes closed, as she imagined Monstris spinning around in these happy colours, as if he were in a magical washing machine.

After a few seconds she moved her hand out from her body, as if she was holding something (she was holding Monstris). She jumped up and was skipping, dancing and laughing, and said, "Mummy, Mummy, can we hang Monstris up to dry now? Then he can hang there and become a really nice and happy Monstris?"

"Sure we can, if you want to do that," I said.

And that is what we did. We pretended to hang Monstris up outside so he could dry in the sun. Then she was a really happy little girl again, ready to play. This whole exercise took only a few minutes, far less than a tantrum would have lasted!

Later that night I got the shock of my life. Natasha had gone to bed and I was just going to go up to check on her. As I quietly went into her room I could see that she was sitting up in bed, cross-legged, with her eyes closed and breathing slowly in and out.

"What are you doing, darling?"

"I am meditating, Mummy."

"Oh, honey, that is great. You are such a good girl. Isn't it time to go to sleep now though?"

"But Mummy, when I meditate all those happy colours come back inside of me."

Words of wisdom from a five-year-old.

Additional information for coaches

In a Transformational NLP Break-Through Session

It can be useful to do Mapping Across at certain times in a Break-Through Session by eliciting the submodalities of the problem state and then eliciting the submodalities of the solution stated during the questioning. Then during the intervention, usually nearer the end, you can map across the submodalities from your client's problem to the submodalities of their solution.

Playing with submodalities

It is useful to learn how to "play" with submodalities. For example, one client wanted to improve her relationship with her husband. At the end of our session I was going to do a Somato-Emotional Drop Down Through (see Transformational NLP Coaching Techniques, pages 199–207) on the body area where she had felt that old blame, accusation and judgment toward her husband. She floated inside her mind and when I asked her what it looked like in there, she said, "Like an old courtroom, with a judge, an accuser, a defendant and me in the middle. It looks really old-fashioned and it is dark and stuffy. It is like an old English court, really stiff and boring."

My instincts told me that the Drop Down Through technique was not the most appropriate with this information and instead I started to play around with the submodalities. So I said, "What would happen if you were to open the curtains to let the light in? And then you open the windows, so the whole room becomes filled with sunshine, light and fresh air."

My client got really excited about this and said, "Yes, and I can fire that old judge and the accuser, everyone in that old courtroom, and instead bring in new staff, fresh-looking, vibrant, young, modern and trendy, all sitting there with the latest computers, wired up to the Internet, working really fast, really efficiently, while having fun together, all helping me to achieve my goals and dreams."

I then asked her, "OK, and is this new team ready for their new task? Are they really, really ready?"

"Sure," my client said.

"OK, so their first task is to put in all their effort, in a fun, humorous, calm, loving way (she had given me these specific resources earlier in the session) in order to help you improve your relationship with your husband. So just instruct them to do this and let me know when you have done that."

My client said, "Oh, wow, they are really getting to work. They are working away at their keyboards, doing research on the Internet and giving me the go-ahead."

"Great, so ask your Unconscious Mind to signal with a 'Yes' signal when it has got all the new integrations, learnings and wisdom it needs for it to be able to assist you in creating a happy, loving and harmonious relationship with your husband."

My client was silent for a few seconds. Then she said smilingly, "Yes, it has done that now [I calibrated a 'Yes' signal from her Unconscious Mind]. And it also wants me to know that all of this already exists within our relationship. I just had to open my eyes and see it."

Anchoring

When I was pregnant with my first child, someone gave me a bottle of perfume. I was wearing this perfume during the first few weeks of pregnancy when I was experiencing nausea and even today, 14 years later, I cannot smell this perfume without feeling nauseous, or any perfumes from the same brand, even though I am not pregnant.

Then, when my first little girl was born, I was absolutely amazed that during her first night when she woke up crying, I only had to place my hand on her back, talk to her in a soothing voice and she immediately calmed down. I realized she was deeply connected with my voice and her feelings of being secure and safe.

In my work as a cranial osteopath I have treated many babies who have experienced difficult births. This means that they often have severe headaches. As I release this pain by applying cranial osteopathic techniques, they often cry. If the mother starts breast-feeding her baby while I give the treatment, the baby calms down, so even though I am treating a very painful area, the peaceful feeling the baby gets from being breast-fed is strong enough to dilute the negative feelings he/she feels as I am treating the painful area. What have I just described? Anchors!

What is an anchor?

An "anchor", in NLP terms, is based on the work of Ivan Pavlov, who did a study in 1904 to find out about the stimulus response pattern in the human nervous system. Initially he experimented on dogs. He put a steak in front of them and, when the dogs started salivating, he rang a bell. He put a steak in front of them again and, when they started salivating, he again rang the bell. After a while the dogs started to salivate just when he rang the bell, without the steaks being put in front of them. He had thereby created an "anchor". Pavlov's study won him the Nobel Prize for physiology, so groundbreaking was this research.

Of course we, as human beings, are also animals and we also create stimulus response patterns in our nervous systems. We call those patterns "anchors". Whenever you are in a heightened state, your nervous system searches around your five senses to find a specific explanation for being in this intense state. When it finds something, it links these two neurologically, so that the external trigger fires off the same state in you, creating the same feeling inside. We as human beings are literally "anchoring machines"; we are anchoring all the time. We anchor certain smells with certain feelings and memories, certain sounds with certain feelings (remember how you used to feel as a child when you heard the ice-cream van chime?), and certain textures with certain inner states. For example, as soon as my youngest daughter sees socks with patterns on them she starts itching – even without putting them on! This makes mornings in our household pretty hard, as it is very difficult to find comfortable socks for her.

In our speech we also have naturally occurring anchors with the way we use our tone of voice. For instance, your tone of voice will go up at the end of a sentence when you are asking a question, and when you are making a statement your tone remains at the same level. When you are issuing a command, your tone goes down at the end of the sentence.

In an experiment shown on the well-known TV programme *Child of our Time*, with Professor Robert Winston, researchers gave a group of English five-year-olds five different types of food and tried to get them to remember the words for these foods in Polish. The kids were given five minutes to learn these words and they could not touch, taste or smell the food, only look at it and hear the words. After the five minutes was up none of the children could remember the Polish words. Then the researchers gave them five new types of food and this time they could taste, smell, touch and look at the food, as well as hearing the Polish words. After five minutes all the children could remember some of the names in Polish. We use our senses to help us remember; a skill that is needed for learning and enabling us to evolve.

Most babies have learnt to associate the smell, voice and touch of their mother with security, so even if the baby can't see the mother in middle of the night, just smelling, hearing and feeling her will soothe him/her within seconds. Similarly a breast-feeding mother will quickly develop an anchor for producing breast milk at the sound of her baby's cry. So here we have an auditory anchor that will trigger a physiological response. There are also a few universal anchors, such as red and green lights. For most people a red light indicates "stop" and a green light "go".

What we are going to learn now is how we can deliberately create anchors that are useful for us and also how to "collapse", or get rid of, negative anchors that we may have created unintentionally, but which are not useful for us. The reason why anchoring is important is because it enables you to gain control over your emotional state.

You are in charge of your own state

Most people think that their state "runs" them, rather than them having the option of putting themselves in the most powerful, most resourceful and optimal state for what they want to do.

An anchor acts as a stimulus response to capture positive resource states from your personal history, linking them to present and future contexts where the resources are needed. It is very useful for controlling your emotional state and in changing your conditioned responses to stimuli that arise in daily life.

Anchoring enables you to tap into the most powerful, positive and resourceful states from your past and fire them off in an instant, whenever you want to be able to be in the state and behave in the way that is going to achieve the best results. Also, anchoring enables us to change anchors that already exist, which we have already set up and which are not working for us.

Why anchoring is useful

1. Anchoring elicits an intense associated state by recalling a vivid past experience.
2. Anchoring provides a unique stimulus as the state reaches peak intensity.

3. Anchoring breaks the state so that the state changes.
4. Anchoring tests the anchor by providing the same stimulus (notice how you go into the state).

Five keys to successful anchoring

1. The person must be in an intense state.
2. The anchor must be applied at the peak of the state.
3. The stimulus used for the anchor must be unique.
4. The anchor must be repeatable.
5. The more the anchor is created the better the anchor.

One of the main skills to develop for anchoring is state elicitation, which is when you bring up a particular physiology and inner state in someone else. Let us look at the main steps involved in this.

State elicitation process and script for anchoring in *someone else*

1. Get into rapport with the person you are going to do this exercise with.
2. Go into the desired state yourself (so if you are going to elicit enthusiasm you have to first go into the state of enthusiasm, so that you are able to pace and lead the other person into this state. If you are calm and quiet yourself, it will be very difficult for the other person to go into a high-energy state, such as enthusiasm, but if you are already in this state you give the other person permission to access this state as well.
3. "Can you remember a time when you were totally_____ [happy, enthusiastic, inspired, loved, confident, or whichever other positive state the client feels is desirable]?"
4. "Can you remember a specific time?" [Look at the person and notice when you see them remembering a specific time in their past when they felt that way. You may well see the state coming up immediately, so apply the anchor straightaway. Don't wait until you have finished reading your script.]
5. "As you go back to that time now, float down inside your body and see what you saw, hear what you heard, notice what you noticed and

really feel the feelings of being totally _____ [happy, enthusiastic, inspired, loved, confident, or whichever other positive state the client feels is desirable]."

6. It's good to keep the anchor applied until you start to see the person coming out of the state and then you release it (usually you hold the anchor for between five and 15 seconds). This is how you elicit a single state for creating an anchor.

All the anchoring processes are built around two anchoring techniques: creating a Single Resource Anchor and creating a Stacked Resource Anchor (see below). In a Single Resource Anchor we just anchor one positive state, whereas in a Stacked Resource Anchor we anchor several states in the same place, so that one trigger will then fire off several different states (as shown below).

Single and Stacked Resource Anchors

Useful states for a Resource Anchor might be: feeling totally loved, totally happy, totally enthusiastic, totally energized, totally fulfilled, totally in tune, totally peaceful, totally compassionate, totally accepting, totally powerful, totally confident or whatever other positive states you would like to have as inner positive resource states. We elicit each of these states in turn and anchor all of them on, for example, the knuckle, or if you are doing it on yourself, by squeezing your thumb and index finger together. You can also stack each state several times, so that you can go to a number of different times when you felt totally loved, totally happy and so on.

Then you can also elicit all the Positive Resources your Unconscious Mind would feel to be useful. You have now created a very powerful Resource Anchor.

For all the following exercises, imagine you are being a coach to yourself, so you literally read the script to yourself. When I do processes on myself I imagine I have a little Angel Coach sitting on my shoulder, saying the script to me, so I follow her instructions. Therefore I will use the word "you" instead of "I".

Exercise for creating a Resource Anchor

Imagine your Angel Coach sitting on your shoulder and he/she saying to you:

1. "Which positive, wonderful resources would it be useful for you to have? Make a list of them, such as feeling totally loved, totally happy, totally energized and so on. Then think now of the first resource.

2. "Can you remember a time when you felt this _____ [specific Positive Resource]? A specific time [think of a specific time]? Now float back to that time, float inside your body, see what you saw, hear what you heard, notice what you noticed and really feel those feelings of _____ [specific Positive Resource]. As soon as you feel those feelings arise inside your body, squeeze your right thumb and right index finger together, creating an anchor. Keep these fingers squeezed. Now double that feeling. Make it 10 times as strong. 100 times as strong. 1,000 times as strong. As soon as the feeling starts to subside, release your anchor, stop squeezing your thumb and index finger."

3. [Now do Step 2 with all the other Positive Resources, one at a time. Release the anchor between each resource state and only squeeze your thumb and index finger together when you feel the feelings of your positive state strongly inside your body.]

4. "We are also going to anchor with the Unconscious Mind, so now ask your Unconscious Mind to provide you with all the resources it feels you need that would be most suitable for you. Your Unconscious Mind is very wise and it knows exactly what it is you need. Just allow these resources to come up inside your body and mind now. As soon as you feel the resources come up within you – as a rush of positive feelings and energy flowing into your body and mind – squeeze your thumb and index finger together. Now double that feeling, make it 10 times as strong, 100 times as strong, 1,000 and a million times as strong. Release the thumb and index finger as soon as you feel the state come off."

You have now created a Resource Anchor. You can use this to help put you in a truly intense, resourceful state, which you can then use to help you through big events, such as giving a presentation, experiencing childbirth, attending a job interview, going on a date. You can also use it to change a negative feeling to a specific trigger, and we do that in the technique called Collapse Anchors (which we will go through soon, see pages 92–4).

Circle of Excellence

We are now going to learn a useful anchoring technique called the Circle of Excellence. This is like a super-intense Resource Anchor, which might be very helpful to use in stressful situations.

Imagine a circle in front of you.

- Now think about which Positive Resources you would like to have in this circle, such as: happiness, energy, love, excitement, enthusiasm, and so on.
- Then imagine your Angel Coach sitting on your shoulder saying to you, "Can you remember a time when you felt total __ [happiness, confidence, love, peace]? A specific time? Great! Float back to that time now, float inside your body and see what you saw, hear what you heard, notice what you noticed and feel those feelings of total _____ [Positive Resource]. As soon as you feel those feelings come up, step inside your circle [so you step inside the circle when you feel them arise inside you]. Now make those feelings doubly strong, 10 times as strong, 100 times as strong, 1,000 times as strong. Then step out of the circle." You step out of the circle as soon as you feel you are coming out of the state. You only want the peak states to be anchored inside the circle, so make sure you calibrate yourself well.
- Now do the same process with all the Positive Resources you want.
- Then also do Unconscious Mind and Higher Self elicitation (you elicit the Higher Self in the same way as you elicit the Unconscious Mind as there is direct communication between them), so your Angel Coach says, "Your Unconscious Mind and Higher Self are very wise and they know exactly all the Positive Resources you need that would be the most useful for you. As soon as you feel these Positive Resources come up inside you, step inside the circle [step

inside the circle as soon as you feel them come up]. Now double that feeling, make it 10 times as strong, 100 times as strong, 1,000 times as strong. Then step out of the circle."

- Ask yourself now which colour you would like to place in the circle and then imagine filling this circle with this positive colour and then step inside the circle and let this positive colour flow into every cell of your being. Step out of the circle.

- Now ask yourself, which phrase would you like to place in the circle, such as, "I can do anything. Go for it! Yippee!" or whatever you feel is most appropriate. Then step inside the circle and scream out this positive phrase.

- Now ask yourself which song you would like to have in the circle. Then step inside your circle and sing that song to yourself, or imagine the song playing really loudly inside your mind, while you dance to it (or if you have the music near by, play it out loud). Step out of the circle.

- Now step inside the circle again and feel and imagine all your Positive Resources coming up inside you, the positive colours, while standing, or even dancing in the circle, singing your song to yourself (or letting it play out loud) and screaming out your positive phrases. You should now go into a really up-beat state. Step out of the circle.

- Now pick up your Circle of Excellence and put it in your back pocket. Whenever you need all these Positive Resources you can just place this circle in front of you and step inside it.

Collapse Anchors

We can use the Collapse Anchors process to get rid of a minor unwanted state that is highly contextualized (which means getting rid of minor unwanted feelings that are triggered in specific contexts). Good examples are: whenever someone looks at you in a particular way that makes you feel bad; whenever your partner speaks to you in a certain tone of voice that makes you get irritable, or whenever you have to get up in front of an audience and feel nervous.

States that are not minor unwanted states are panic, terror, obsession and fear. The state also has to be *contextualized*, so that if someone has depression and you then ask them when they experience this, and they say all the time, then that is not a minor unwanted state and it is not contextualized, since they do it all the time, so, in other words, they do it everywhere.

During my practitioner training, my trainer, David Shepherd, demonstrated this process on me. I would go into a particular negative state every time I heard my father use a certain tone of voice on the phone. But after the demonstration, I never experienced this negative state in relation to my father again; I was fine with him on the phone and I was also fine with him in person. It did not matter whether he used that tone again – I was still fine inside and the external trigger never fired off the same state again. Instead I just felt happy and peaceful. Weird and true! Thank you, David!

Collapse Anchors can be a really quick fix.

Doing the Collapse Anchors exercise on yourself

You have already created a Resource Anchor with your thumb and index finger and also your own Circle of Excellence. Make sure both of these produce a highly intense Positive Resource state within you – if you have not done those exercises recently, do them now!

Great! What I want you to do now is to think about something that causes you to go into a minor unwanted state or a behaviour that is highly contextualized. Perhaps it is someone's tone of voice, or the way someone looks at you, or even a particular thought. Whatever it is, find it now and feel yourself going into that negative state. Good. Then break that negative state by moving your body and "shaking" the state off.

Just check now that the positive state produced by your Resource Anchor and Circle of Excellence is much more intense (positive) than the negative state you want to remove. So the intensity should be stronger on the positive than on the negative. If you feel that the positive is not stronger than the negative, then you have to "juice up" (intensify) your Resource Anchor and Circle of Excellence, as it *has to be more intense* than the negative state you want to get rid of. Once that is done you proceed as follows.

Now think again of the thing that causes you to go into a minor unwanted state or behaviour and feel yourself go into the negative state.

Imagine your Circle of Excellence in front of you and step inside it. Feel all those Positive Resources come up within you, make them even stronger, fill the circle with your positive colour and positive phrase, play your song out loud if you can, otherwise imagine it playing in your head, and now also fire off your Positive Resource Anchor with your right thumb and index finger and feel all those Positive Resources come up within you as well.

What you should feel happening now is that your wonderful Positive Resources are so much stronger than your negative state that they totally collapse the negative state; instead you are just filled with your Positive Resources.

Still remaining inside your Circle of Excellence and still squeezing your Resource Anchor, imagine how you can go out into the future and notice how differently you are able to deal with situations that in the past used to trigger your old unwanted state. Now you fill your future with all your Positive Resources and notice how different you are able to be. Then come back to the present moment.

You have now linked your initial trigger, which used to trigger your old negative state, with your Positive Resources! Well done!

Chapter 5
Advanced-Level Techniques of Transformational NLP

Healing with the Highest Intention Reframe

This is a wonderful process to perform as you have direct communication with the Unconscious Mind. You have to be very good at calibrating your own Unconscious Mind's "Yes" and "No" signals, so you can detect the *real* "Yes" and "No" and not what you *think* the real "Yes" and "No" is. Although the technique in itself is really easy, it is this exquisite calibration that causes the Healing with the Highest Intention Reframe to be in the advanced section. This technique has its roots in the Six-Step Reframe (a well-known orthodox NLP process), but I have changed it quite a bit, so therefore I have given it this new name.

Case studies

One woman I was working with had developed a cancerous secondary tumour. I first calibrated her Unconscious Mind's "Yes" and "No" signals and there were distinct differences. As I started to do the Healing with the Highest Intention Reframe I kept asking her Unconscious Mind what the highest intention of this growth was. After a while she started to say things like, "To learn to love myself." I then asked, "Is that the highest intention?" My client said, "Yes", but her physiology gave me a "No" signal. So I asked her, "What is the highest intention of 'To learn to love myself'?" She then answered, "To continue the growth, whatever the growth is." I then asked if that was the highest intention and both my client and her physiology said, "Yes." If I had not used my calibration skills I would have thought that the highest intention

95

of the secondary tumour was to learn to love herself (which my client also believed it was), while in fact it was instead to *continue the growth, whatever the growth is*.

Since my client had been diagnosed with this tumour, she had embarked on a journey of self-discovery and spiritual growth and the secondary tumour growth was forcing her to continue her spiritual growth. It was literally a physical metaphor of the highest intention.

My client had a strong tendency to try to be dependent on others and make herself helpless, so others would help her. She would often ask me to tell her what I thought she should do, which I refused to do, since that would have been to play into her pattern of disempowering herself. Instead I took her through processes where she herself had to come up with the solutions, learnings and insights that would help her to grow in wisdom. Her tumour started to shrink within a few months of her session.

A man I worked with had developed knee pain and had all the symptoms of a meniscus injury. Several years before he'd had a previous meniscus injury on this same knee, which needed an operation. My client was convinced that he needed an operation on his knee again, but decided to try to see if NLP could help him before he decided one way or the other. I did a Healing with the Highest Intention Reframe on his knee and within a few weeks the pain had disappeared. The highest intention for the knee pain was to follow his own path and as his Unconscious Mind found new positive ways of doing this, the pain in the knee disappeared and he never needed an operation.

I did the same technique on a young girl who had a stubborn wart on her knee. It had initially gone a year earlier after she fell and scraped it off, but now it had grown back. This wart was the size of two large raisins. I did a Healing with the Highest Intention Reframe on the girl and the wart disappeared within a few months and has never grown back. The highest intention for the wart was to teach the girl to love herself just the way she was and that it is OK for her to be different, and as her Unconscious Mind found new ways of still fulfilling this highest intention the wart could start to disappear. Weird and true!

The beauty of Healing with the Highest Intention Reframe is that you gain access to the Unconscious Mind by calibrating the "Yes" and

"No" signals. The Unconscious Mind has full access to the Spirit, to the Higher Consciousness, but it might not always be fully aware of the very highest intention from the highest spiritual realms. So by asking for the highest intention you are able to find the highest intention also from a spiritual level, and then you are able to bring that down into the unconscious level so that the Unconscious Mind is better able to understand and integrate fully what is required of it. This is a very powerful exercise. You can still do this exercise and get tremendous benefits from it even if you are unsure of your own Unconscious Mind signals.

Outline of process

Before you start

• Find the behaviour/physiological issue to be changed (such as back pain, headache, migraine, sinus problems, relationship issues, problems with money or tiredness).

• Find your Unconscious Mind "Yes" and "No" signals (see pages 38–40).

Process

Imagine your Angel Coach saying to you, "I would now like to ask your Unconscious Mind, what is the highest intention of this _____ [behaviour/physiological issue to be changed].

"What is the highest intention of that?

"What is the highest intention of that?"

Your Angel Coach keeps asking for the highest intention until you feel you have found the exact highest intention. When you think you have found it your Angel Coach asks you, "Is that the highest intention for you?"

Here check with your Unconscious Mind whether this is the highest intention. If you get a "No" here then your Angel Coach keeps asking for the highest intention until you know you have found the right one and your Unconscious Mind confirms this with a "Yes" signal.

Once you have found the highest intention your Angel Coach asks you, "I would now like you to find three, five, 10 or more new Positive Behaviours that will fulfil this highest intention of _____ [whatever your highest intention was] while still remaining in alignment with the healing work we are doing. What are these alternative Positive Behaviours?"

Here you state what these alternative Positive Behaviours are.

Your Angel Coach now says, "I would now like to ask your Unconscious Mind, do you understand?" (You have to get a "Yes" signal from your Unconscious Mind).

"Are you willing to take responsibility for implementing this change now?" (You have to get a "Yes" signal from your Unconscious Mind).

"Is there anything your Unconscious Mind wants your Conscious Mind to know?"

"I now want you to instruct your Unconscious Mind to start this change now."

If at any point (when asking, "Do you understand? Are you willing to take responsibility?") you get a "No" signal from your Unconscious Mind, your Angel Coach asks you the following reframe questions:

- Ask your Unconscious Mind what the Positive Learnings are for you, Positive Learnings that will help you to understand/take responsibility for this now?
- What is it that your Unconscious Mind wants you to know and learn, the knowing and learning which will help you to understand/ take responsibility for this now?
- What do you need to pay attention to so you can do that?
- What do you need to focus on so you can do that now?

Once you have replied, your Angel Coach continues with the normal script. These reframe questions help your Unconscious Mind to be in full alignment with the healing work you are doing.

Additional information for coaches

You have to calibrate in all the main representational systems – Visual, Auditory and Kinaesthetic. Some coaches ask their client to answer "Yes" and "No" with finger signals, which is common practice in hypnosis. But clients might "fake" these finger signals (that is, their Conscious Mind will think it is a "Yes" signal and move the "Yes" finger), while if you are able to calibrate the client's Unconscious Mind's "Yes" and "No" signals exquisitely well, then the client cannot fool you. You also do not need the client to go into a deep trance in order for you to be able to calibrate their "Yes" and "No" signals, so it is easier to do for you to do during coaching (once you have developed your calibration skills).

An example of the Healing with the Highest Intention Reframe in action

Coach: "So Anne, let's imagine you are looking at yourself from more of a distance [pointing to somewhere on the floor]. Is there a behaviour or physiological condition that Anne does that she would like to change?"

Anne: "Yes, I would like to change the fact that I never look after my health and therefore I am putting on weight."

Coach: "Is it OK if I speak to Anne's Unconscious Mind about this?"

Anne: "Yes."

Coach: "Great. So what is the highest intention of this behaviour of *never looking after your health, so therefore you put on weight?*"

Anne: "To punish me."

Coach: "What is the highest intention of *to punish me?*"

Anne: "To hurt me."

Coach: "What is the highest intention of *to hurt me?*"

Anne: "To cause me to change."

Coach: "What is the highest intention of *to cause me to change?*"

Anne: "So that I grow."

Coach: "What is the highest intention of *so that I grow?*"

Anne; "So I can be all that I am meant to be."

Coach: "Is that the highest intention?"

Anne: "No."

Coach: "So what is the highest intention of *so that I can be all that I am meant to be?*"

Anne: "So I can be of service."

Coach: "Is that the highest intention?"

Anne: "Yes" (coach calibrates a "No" signal from Unconscious Mind).

Coach: "What is the highest intention of *so that I can be of service?*"

Anne: "To help the world grow in love."

Coach: "Is that the highest intention?"

Anne: "So that I grow in love, and from my love I can help the world grow in love."

Coach: "Is that the highest intention?"

Anne: "Yes" (coach still calibrating a "No" signal).

Coach: "So what is the highest intention of *so that I grow in love and from my love I can help the world grow in love?*"

Anne: "To be love, so the world can grow in love."

Coach: "Is that the highest intention?"

Anne: "Yes" (coach calibrating a "Yes" signal).

Coach: "Great, so I now would like to ask your Unconscious Mind to come up with three, five, 10 or an infinite number of alternative Positive Behaviours that would still satisfy this highest intention of *to be love, so the world can grow in love*, while being in alignment with the healing work we are doing here today."

Anne remained silent for a little while and then said, "To meditate every day, to show my family how much I love them, to stop and experience the beauty in my life, to give thanks for everything I have in my life – every day. To write a gratitude journal, to focus on the positive instead of the negative, to tell my body how much I love it, to do gentle exercise every day, to make my own vegetable and fruit juices and to eat organic food as much as possible so that my body gets proper nourishment, to focus on my body being my physical temple, allowing me to experience life and to focus more on the divinity within my body rather than on how it looks physically, to realize my husband loves me – the Spirit living inside of me – and that this is more important than the way I look."

Coach: "I now would like to ask your Unconscious Mind, does it understand?"

Anne: "Yes" (coach calibrating a "No" signal).

Coach: "Ask your Unconscious Mind, what are the Positive Learnings that would allow you to understand this now?"

Anne: "That I have the power within me to look after myself and the more I look after myself the more I am able to look after others."

Coach: "What would your Unconscious Mind want you to know and learn so that you can understand this now?"

Anne: "That I am loved just the way I am and the more I love myself, the healthier my body is."

Coach: "Ask your Unconscious Mind what it wants you to pay attention to, so that you can understand this now?"

Anne: "That I do understand. It is quite simple, really."

Coach: "I would now like to ask your Unconscious Mind, does it understand?"

Anne: "Yes" (coach calibrating a "Yes" signal from the Unconscious Mind).

Coach: "Is it willing to accept responsibility for implementing this change now?"

Anne: "Yes" (coach calibrating a "Yes" signal).

Coach: "Is there anything your Unconscious Mind wants your Conscious Mind to know?"

Anne: "Yes. To know that the more I look after myself, the more love I will feel inside, and from this love the world can grow, instead of my body growing."

Coach: "Great. I now want you to instruct your Unconscious Mind to set up this change now and to signal with a 'Yes' signal when it has done that."

Anne: "Yes" (coach calibrating a "Yes" signal).

Parts Integration

A woman came to see me some years ago because she desperately wanted to have a baby. She was happily married and she and her husband had being trying for a baby for nearly eight years. The problem was that she felt she already had a baby – her business. She had been nurturing her business for a long time and she was very successful, with several employees. On one hand she felt that she wanted a baby and on the other that her business was her baby. She believed that she could not have both. As we looked for the highest intention (called "chunking up", see page 109) on these supposedly conflicting thoughts she realized that both "parts" of the conflict (baby and business) had as their highest intention for her to be happy and fulfilled.

Once she had solved this inner conflict she was able to make the changes she needed to in her business so that it was all right for her to take the time off to make room in her life for a real-life baby. She is now the proud mother of a little boy and her business is still flourishing.

When I was a teenager I used to help out at a local zoo and one spring we were sent a beautiful little baby adder. The problem for this baby snake was that it had two heads. I had never seen a two-headed, conjoined snake before! Because the two heads were the same size they would quarrel about which head ate first and as soon as one head tried to eat, the other would attack it and vice versa. The result was a starving baby snake. If this snake was going to live a long, happy life the two heads would have to learn to get on and realize that they both had the same highest intention: to give nourishment to the snake, so that it could enjoy life.

What I have just described is a type of Parts Conflicts. These conflicts are literally when you have different aspects within yourself going in different directions. You might have one positive part wanting you to do something, say for example, to start a new career, and another negative part wanting you to stay where you are now, because perhaps you might fail if you tried something new. These negative inner conflicts can become very destructive and it is important to heal them, so that they become whole with the wholeness within you. This wholeness within you is your Divine Source.

You can have many different types of conflicts, such as:

Internal conflicts
- A part of me wants X and another part wants Y (toward/toward conflict).
- I feel as though I am being pulled apart.
- I am torn in two directions.
- On the one hand X, and on the other hand Y.
- A part of me says it is not all right to do X, Y and Z.
- Toward/away from conflict.

Incongruent behaviour
- I don't know why I did it; it's just not me.
- I don't know why I did it; I just wasn't myself.

Sequential incongruence
- One minute I'm happy, the next I'm sad, and I don't know why.
- The alcoholic who wants to give up drinking. One minute he is congruent about giving up, the next he is congruent about drinking.

Part-time problems
When you sometimes think you can do something and at other times think you cannot.

Addictive behaviour
Any addictive behaviour, such as being addicted to alcohol, cigarettes, food, gambling, obsessive thought patterns, obsessive compulsive disorder and so on, are all an indication of a Parts Conflict.

I have also found that if someone carries out a particular behaviour a lot, they often have a Parts Conflict. It is as if they have developed an addiction to this particular behaviour – a particular thought pattern. Common addictive behaviours I have seen are: depression, anxiety, panic, confusion, avoiding responsibility, blame, anger, letting go of a problem then picking it up again, only to let it go – and then picking it up again.

The way you resolve a Parts Conflict is actually quite similar to a Healing with the Highest Intention Reframe (see pages 99–101), just that here you apply it to both parts in conflict with each other – the "good" one and the "bad" one.

Simple outline of Parts Integration process

1. Find the conflict.
2. Place your hands, palms facing up, in front of you.
3. Ask the Problem Part to come out on one hand (imagine you have the "bad" part coming out onto one of your hands). Find Visual, Auditory, Kinaesthetic.
4. Ask the opposite part to come out on the other hand. Find Visual, Auditory, Kinaesthetic.
5. Ask the Problem Part: What is the highest intention of this behaviour? What is the highest intention of that? Keep asking until you find the highest intention. Confirm with the Unconscious Mind.

6. Ask the opposite part what its highest intention is. Keep asking until you reach the same, or very similar, highest intention as for the Problem Part. Confirm with the Unconscious Mind.

7. Ask the parts if they realize that they both have the same highest intention and if it would be easier for them to fulfil their highest intention for you by working together. Ask them if they both have positive qualities the other one could benefit from. Ask the parts to realize whether they were once part of a larger whole and if they would like to become whole once again.

8. Notice the hands coming together as the two parts want to work together now. Imagine you are taking both parts inside your heart and integrating them.

9. Then go out into the future to the Chamber of Treasures, where you receive a gift that will help you with all of this and then come back to now.

Parts Integration exercise

Imagine that your Angel Coach asks you, "So how is this a problem? How is this a conflict?" She keeps asking these questions until you feel you have identified the Parts Conflict.

Your Angel Coach instructs you to hold your hands, palms up, in front of you, but to make sure that your elbows are not resting on anything, so that they are free in space.

Your Angel Coach now asks, "I would now like the Problem Part to come out on one hand. Which hand does this Part like to come out onto?" Wait until you notice which hand it prefers to come out onto.

Then your Angel Coach says, "Does this Part have a shape, colour, feeling or sound?"

Notice what it feels, sounds and looks like.

Then your Angel Coach says, "I now want the opposite Part to come out on the other hand. What does this Part look, sound and feel like?"

Just notice what this Part looks, sounds and feels like.

Your Angel Coach asks, "I would now like to ask the Problem Part, what is your highest intention? What is the highest intention of that?"

Your Angel Coach keeps asking this until you feel you have reached the highest intention. She then asks, "Is that the highest intention for you?"

Here you must ask your Unconscious Mind to confirm that this is the highest intention. If you get a "No", then your Angel Coach keeps asking for the highest intention. If you are uncertain about your Unconscious Mind signals, then just keep asking for the highest intention until you get to the intention where you can feel a shift inside you.

Your Angel Coach now asks, "I would now like to ask the opposite Part, what is your highest intention? What is the highest intention of that?"

Your Angel Coach keeps asking this until you reach the same or very similar highest positive intention as the Problem Part got to. (Ask the Unconscious Mind to confirm that this is the highest positive intention or that you just feel instinctively it is the right one.)

Your Angel Coach now says, "Can both Parts realize that they both have the same highest intention for you? Would it now be easier for them to fulfil their highest intention by working together? Does each Part have any positive qualities the other Part could benefit from? Do both Parts realize that they were once part of a larger whole? Would they like to become whole once again? Have you noticed how your hands are coming together all by themselves as the Parts realize how much easier it would be for them to fulfil their highest intention for you if they were to work together?

"How would it be if you were to allow both Parts to merge and then to take them inside your heart now?"

Once you feel that both Parts have merged and you have taken them inside your heart, your Angel Coach says, "Now go out into the future, and see, hear and feel how you are able to fulfil this highest intention of _____ [the highest intention both Parts had in your life] as they are now working together and notice how this _____ [highest intention] flows inside every day of your future life, and notice how different you are now. Go out all the way to eternity now and there visit your own unique Chamber of Treasures, where your most Evolved Wise Self meets you. You step inside this chamber and your Evolved Wise Self gives you a treasure – a gift – for having done this work on yourself. This gift will help you on your journey through life. Notice what this gift is. What does it represent to you? Then take this gift and sprinkle the essence of this gift and what it represents to you into every day of your life, from eternity all the way back to now and feel how it is helping you fulfil this highest intention of _____ [the Parts' highest intention], all the way back to now."

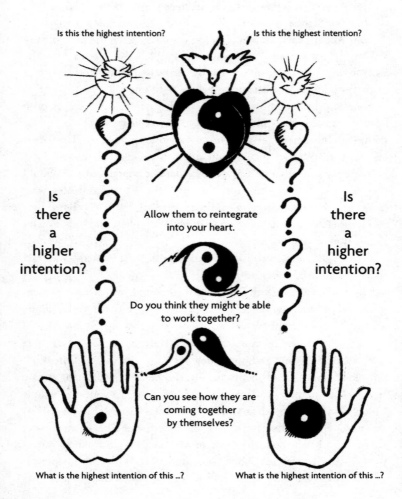

Is this the highest intention?　　Is this the highest intention?

Is there a higher intention?

Allow them to reintegrate into your heart.

Do you think they might be able to work together?

Is there a higher intention?

Can you see how they are coming together by themselves?

What is the highest intention of this ...?　　What is the highest intention of this ...?

Chapter 6
Logical Levels

When you are working on yourself or with others, you want to find the highest Logical Level of the problem, so that when you release it, you release the deepest structure of the problem; that is you remove it completely, together with its roots, so that it cannot grow back again (unless you choose to plant new seeds of the original problem-thought pattern – not something that is recommended).

For example, one businesswoman I saw believed that she was evil, which caused her to shut out everyone she loved, because she tried to protect them from herself. As she released this belief she went back to the womb to a time when her mother was eight months pregnant with her and she heard her say that she wanted to get rid of this "awful lump" (remember to see the event only as a metaphor that the client's Unconscious Mind is presenting to her, so that she can receive the learnings she needs in order to heal this – it is not necessarily something that has actually happened). My client felt that her mother wanted to get rid of her and she got extremely angry with her and closed her heart to her. As she closed her heart she formed the belief that she was evil, since only evil people close their hearts.

When we released this Limiting Belief, all the other smaller Limiting Beliefs were released as well, because they were all linked to this main Limiting Belief, which for this client was the lynchpin, the "monster fish", that was the root cause of her presenting problem. This was her Highest Logical Level of the problem. The only way to know you have found the Highest Logical Level of the problem is to calibrate your client.

How to find the Limiting Belief

In NLP we aim to work with the higher-level presenting problem, since that will allow many other lower-level presenting problems to change, too, just as it did with my client. Usually, the highest-level presenting problem is the major Limiting Belief or Limiting Decision we have, or the main Problem Strategy, or even a major metaphor, which if it is released all the other problems start to disappear as well. Sometimes you will find this highest level during your normal questions, but there is also a particular "chasing down" question you can ask, which seems to be able to draw that major "deep fish" out. And the question is:

"If I were to imagine I could see myself and my life over there (pointing to somewhere on the floor), what is it that I believe deep down that I am, or what is it that I believe about myself or about life that is causing all these problems?"

You then answer this – for example, "I am not good enough". Then you ask, "So what am I or what do I believe about myself or about life that is causing me to believe I am not good enough?"

Keep asking this with whatever answer you get. This is a very uncomfortable exercise, by the way, but it only takes a few minutes (never longer than five minutes, although it might feel a lot longer).

Doing this process will start to give you the lynchpin, that big, big fish, and you really need to find one in order for you to create maximum change in your life.

Then you need to see which of the monster fish you have found is the lynchpin, the one which if it disappeared all the others would disappear, too. You can do this by listing them all and asking yourself which is the main one. Then in your intervention you will make sure all the ones you have diagnosed are released, starting with the one you said was the major one. You will, however, not know which one was really the biggest until the intervention – by noticing which one creates the biggest shift in you.

You also have to be aware of not phrasing a negative Limiting Belief such as, "I'm not good enough", because the Unconscious Mind can't compute a negative – what it will hear is that it is good enough. What I usually ask here is, "So what are you that is causing you to believe you are not good enough?" Keep asking this question until you get the big fish that you need; the highest Logical Level of the problem. Common examples are things like, "I'm unlovable", "I'm worthless",

"I'm a failure", "I'm nothing", and it can also be a metaphor, such as one woman seeing her depression as a giant squid that was suffocating her, or a man who felt that he had this beast inside and this was the lynchpin of the main problem.

We are discussing Logical Levels before we move into the linguistic part of the book (see pages 124–70) as it is important to understand that you always guide your questioning from a Higher Logical Level. You want to be able to see the Higher Logical Level of how someone, including yourself, has developed the problem, and then use your questions to find the root thought structures, such as the Limiting Beliefs, values and Negative Thought patterns, which start to lead you to the lynchpin of the problem, which is the Higher Logical Level of the presenting problem.

Logical Levels in chunking

Chunking up

Sometimes we drown in the details of a problem and then it is useful to come up for air and see the bigger picture. Here we use "chunking up" questions, which take us to a higher level, making it easier to see things more clearly.

We can chunk up by asking questions such as:

"What is the highest intention of this?"
"For what purpose?"
"What does this mean?"
"What's the bigger picture?"
"What is this an example of?"

Here you are also looking for the pattern of the problem, the Higher Logical Level of the problem, and you guide your questions (both chunking up and down) in such a way that you are able to find the structure of the problem pattern, which will lead you to the monster fish. In this way you keep a Higher Logical Level awareness of the problem during your whole questioning session.

Chunking down

Sometimes we can get stuck with big ideas, grand plans and great visions, without being able to see how we can manifest them in reality. And we can, of course, get stuck into thinking that everything is awful and everyone is horrible, and it is, of course, always everyone else's fault that our lives are the way they are. When we do this we are unable to see how we ourselves create our experience due to our specific thought structures and behaviours.

Often it is useful to start by getting the bigger picture before you dive into the detail. Chunking down is a way of fishing for more details, more data and more specifics about the high-level information you already have. You chunk down by asking questions such as,

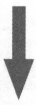

"How did you that?" "When do you do that?"
"What specifically?" "What are examples of this?"
"What is the root cause of all this?"
"What are the various Problem Strategies, Parts Conflicts?"
"Are there any Limiting Beliefs and Limiting Decisions?"
See also Meta Model (pages 125–8) questions.

Up and down

You can use both methods together as a way of cutting through the maze of a problem, so that you are able to diagnose its specific features (chunking down), while also being able to see its overall pattern (chunking up).

Logical Levels for presenting problems

The paradox

The paradox in this is that you find the Highest Logical Level of the problem when you drill deep down into its structure – by finding the Problem Strategies, deeply held Limiting Beliefs and Negative Thoughts, and the Highest Logical Level of these will be that unconscious structure (a thought, Problem Strategy, Limiting Belief, metaphor) that, when released, will release all the other lower-level problems, too. So you do not find the Highest Logical Level of the problem by chunking up, but by drilling deep down! This is the paradox.

Highest level

When that highest-level monster fish is released all the other problems will go as well. This could be a major Limiting Belief or Limiting Decision, or a deep metaphor. Some typical ones I have encountered are, "I am worthless", "I am bad", "I am evil", "I am a monster", "I am unlovable", but I have also encountered metaphors such as a snake, a deathly fog, a grey stone, a poison, a dark shadow, a snake pit and so on. The only way you will know that this is the highest level of the problem structure is to calibrate it for your client. You can also ask the Unconscious Mind and calibrate the "Yes" and "No" signals.

Never assume the monster fish is a particular fish. Each and every one of us is unique and just because you might have previously experienced a monster fish to be, "I am unlovable" it does not mean that this is the monster fish every time. Always keep an open mind and use your calibration skills at all times.

Lower levels

There are lots of examples of "problems" that may not seem to be connected, but when you start to really drill deep into them you start to notice a pattern emerging. If you are working with someone else they may not be consciously aware of this pattern when you start to notice it yourself. Refrain from telling them and instead guide your questions so that the person becomes aware through his/her own discoveries.

Chapter 7
The Inner Structure
and Programming

Strategies

When we experience problems in our lives, it will be because we have a strategy for performing that problem. It is necessary that we find the strategy for how we perform a problem, and it is also necessary to find the strategy for how we know the problem has gone.

You later release the Problem Strategy with the Higher-Self Healing process (outlined on pages 195–99). At the end of a healing coaching session you ensure that you are now performing the strategy for knowing how the problem has gone (Solution Strategy). If you are performing it for someone else, you can cement this further by taking the person through a meditation at the end, which also includes their Solution Strategy as part of the meditation (see Final Meditation in Chapter 18, pages 250–53).

What is a strategy?

A strategy is the sequence of internal and external representations leading to a specific outcome. We have a strategy for every behaviour we carry out.

Why is it useful to know about strategies?

By knowing your own strategy, for instance for carrying out a problem, you can release it more easily. Also by knowing what the Solution Strategy is you can let your Unconscious Mind know that the problem has gone.

If you want to be creative, then learn what your Creative Strategy is. If you know your strategies for understanding and learning then, when you want to understand and learn something, you can go through the order and sequence of your understanding and learning strategies to enable you to attain those states far more rapidly.

To elicit strategies easily, quickly and accurately you need to learn the following:

- Chunking – most behaviours are composed of chunks that are too big, so we need to break the behaviour down into individual elements.
- Being able to discover the order and sequence of the components of the strategy within those particular elements.
- Knowing when a person is actually relating the real Problem Strategy to you and not just analyzing it.

Here is a simplified strategy elicitation, useful for eliciting Problem Strategies. Imagine your Angel Coach saying,

1. "Can you remember a time when you did _____ ?"
2. "A specific time?"
3. "Great, so float back to that time now, float inside your body. See what you saw, hear what you heard, feel what you felt and notice what you noticed. What is the first thing that happens? Do you get a feeling? Do you see a picture? Do you say something to yourself? What is the very first thing that happens?"
4. "So after you have _____ [what you just said], what is the next thing that happens? Do you get a picture? Do you say something to yourself? Do you get a feeling?"

Keep repeating Step 4 until you notice you exit the strategy and enter straight into the problem. Also be aware of loops – that is, when you are recycling the strategy.

Always make sure that you, at some point, get a Kinaesthetic component and when you do, let your Angel Coach ask you, "Where do you feel that?" If you get a feeling, without specifying what type of feeling it is, make sure you find out which type of feeling, so your Angel Coach asks, "What type of feeling is it?" I always do this bit, since I have noticed that when I am able to specify the feeling and where it is, then it is easier for the Unconscious Mind to know the *exact structure* of what it is we want to release later on, when we release the Problem Strategy. Always write down the strategy word for word, the way you say it, or if you are working with someone else, the way the person says it – and not how you should say it grammatically.

Here is an example of a strategy elicitation (the presenting problem here was a client's depression). Remember to also be aware of the person's physiology as they say their strategy.

- "Can you remember a time when you did that?" (The client knew I meant her depression). Client nods her head.
- "A specific time?" Client nods her head again.
- "Great, so float back to that time now, float inside your body. See what you saw, hear what you heard, feel what you felt and notice what you noticed. What is the first thing that happens? Do you get a feeling? Do you see a picture? Do you say something to yourself? What is the very first thing that happens?"
- Client, "**I feel this overwhelming sadness**" (she places her right hand over her heart).
- "Where?"
- "In my heart."
- "OK, so after you feel this overwhelming sadness, what is the next thing that happens? Do you get a picture? Do you say something to yourself? Do you get a feeling?"
- "**It is all black, like a giant mass of blackness suffocating me**" (both hands go up to her throat).
- "Where do you feel that?"
- "My throat."
- "OK, so after you feel this blackness, like a giant mass of blackness suffocating you, what is the next thing that happens? Do you get a picture? Do you say something to yourself? Do you get a feeling?"
- "Then I just cry and cry all day." (She has now already exited by going into the Problem Behaviour, so this is not part of her strategy to get there.)

So her Problem Strategy is the following:

"**I feel this overwhelming sadness** [right hand touching heart], **it is all black, like a giant mass of blackness suffocating me** [both hands going up to throat]."

When I read this back to her, I read only her words, but I mimicked her physiology with my own physiology (given in square brackets).

Now find out your own Problem Strategy for doing a particular problem in your life. Once you have found the problem, imagine you have your Angel Coach sitting on your shoulder asking you the following:

- "Can you remember a time when you did that?"
- "A specific time?"
- "Good. So float back to that time, float inside your body, see what you saw, hear what you heard, feel what you felt and notice what you noticed. What is the first thing that happens? Do you get a feeling? Do you see a picture? Do you say something to yourself? What is the very first thing that happens?"
- "And after that _____ [whatever you answered], what is the next thing that happens? Do you get a picture? Do you get a feeling? Do you say something to yourself? What is the next thing that happens?"
- "And after that _____ [whatever you answered], what is the next thing that happens?" (You keep asking this question until you exit. That is, you go into the Problem State.)

Now write down your Problem Strategy here:

_____

_____

Be aware that a Problem Strategy is usually very short, since it is highly effective – otherwise it would not have created a problem for you.

Solution Strategy

Now let us find your Solution Strategy. Imagine your Angel Coach sitting on your shoulder asking you the following questions:

"If I were to have a magic wand, so that this problem was gone, how would you know that it had gone?", "What would you see?", "What would you hear?", "What would you notice?", "What would you say to yourself?", "What would you feel?", "How would you be different?"

Write your Solution Strategy down here:

_____

_____

Once we move into the Break-Through process in Part 5 (see pages 188–220), knowing how to find your Problem Strategies and your Solution Strategy will become very useful.

Forming our Inner Screening System

Our Inner Screening System consists of our values, beliefs and past experiences. Therefore it is important to find out your values in the problem area in your life, as you then start to uncover it. You then will re-elicit the values at the end to make sure the Inner Screening System has indeed changed. It also acts as a "convincer" (so that the Unconscious Mind can let go of the doubt and instead become convinced) that change has actually taken place.

Values

A value is a "hot button" that drives a behaviour. Whatever you do is done in order to fulfil a value – even though you are unlikely to be consciously aware of it.

Everything you do serves to fulfil your inner values. For example, you keep your cool with your kids even when they are screaming and hitting each other, because you have a value of always treating them with respect and of wanting to show them, through your behaviour, what is acceptable and what is not.

You do what you do to either move toward pleasurable feelings or values or to move away from, or avoid, painful values or feelings. In NLP the pain values are called Away-From Values and the pleasure values are called Toward Values. This is also what Buddha taught – that everything we do is due to us wanting to move away from pain, toward pleasure and his way of liberating his psyche from this was to learn to just observe the feelings and thoughts inside, because they too would pass. In this way he learnt to detach himself from his reactions to pain or pleasure.

I do not think so much in terms of "away from" or "toward", but rather as "positive energy" or "negative energy". When we give 100 per cent positive energy (positive thoughts and feelings) to a value, that value will work well for us. When we give 100 per cent negative energy to a value, that value will not work well for us. In fact, we will have created a problem in that area of our lives. A metaphor I use in my own mind to look at this is the following. When we are filled with negative thoughts and feelings, our ego has managed to get its claws into us (read more about the ego in Chapter 14, see pages 180–85), and this will lead to conflict, pain and problems, because we are then following the ego's advice in how to lead our lives.

When we are instead filled with positive thoughts and energy we are linked with our Wise Soul and this will create happiness, love and joy in our lives, because we are following our Soul's advice in how to lead our lives.

Our values are rather like portals into our inner drives. But which guide will we follow? The ego or our Soul? Fear or love? Which source of energy will we use to create our lives? When we use the ego's energy we will create more darkness and pain, and when we use our Divine Soul's energy we will create more light, love and happiness.

You can have a mixture of the two energies, such as on this scale:

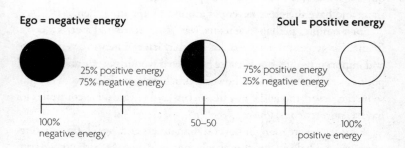

Ego = negative energy **Soul = positive energy**

25% positive energy
75% negative energy

75% positive energy
25% negative energy

100%
negative energy

50–50

100%
positive energy

We are the portals through which this energy flows and our values can help us find out exactly which areas we are allowing divine light energy to flow into and which areas we are letting negative energy flow into. Knowing this enables us to heal and change this, so we can fill our lives, and therefore the world around us, with our divine beauty and light.

When clients come to see me and an area of their lives is not going well, I know their values in that area will be strongly negative. If they are not, then either that area of their lives is not as bad as they suppose, and the problem lies elsewhere, or they are kidding themselves – wanting things to appear better than they actually are.

Values and beliefs form the filters through which we perceive our reality, but beliefs can be better known to the Conscious Mind (apart from the very deep Limiting Beliefs, the big fish, which are always embedded deeply in the Unconscious Mind).

Values can change in an instant and this is a common experience. For example, many of my clients have their life values changed completely when they have a baby. In that instant, as that little baby arrives into the world, the parents take one look at him or her and realize that all their inner values have changed. Suddenly what they thought was important before does not seem so important any more. It is the same with clients who have, or have had, a life-threatening illness. This has brought about a major shift in life values for many of them.

Most of our values were established many years ago. Many were laid down when we were very young, yet they are still likely to be driving our behaviours decades later – simply because we do not know about them and have therefore never got around to updating them.

For example, perhaps someone was poor as a child but is now a financially successful businessman. He may have money as a very strong and important value, but because he still has wounds inside about being poor as a child, he feels that however much he earns it is never enough, so he can never stop and enjoy his success and rewards. He continues to have a "poverty consciousness".

Some values are more important than others and, again, this ranking of values is likely to be completely unconscious. As a result we can spend lots of time, energy and money attempting to fulfil a value that has relatively little importance, while ignoring ones that should be much higher on our list. This is a very common phenomenon.

Because values are associated with worth, meaning and desire, they are a primary source of motivation in people's lives. When people's values are met or matched, they feel a sense of satisfaction, harmony or rapport. When their values are not met or matched, people often feel dissatisfied, incongruent or violated.

How do we elicit values?

Step 1: Finding out the values for a specific area of our lives
(These include: family, relationship, work, personal development, health or spiritual development)

Imagine your Angel Coach sitting on your shoulder asking you,

"What is important to you about _____ [one specific area of life in the list above]?"

For example, "What is important to you about relationships?" "What else is important to you about relationships?" "What else is important to you?" Keep asking this until you have about eight or 10 values. Then your Angel Coach will ask you to number these values from one to eight in order of importance. So your Angel Coach will ask, "Out of these values, which is the most important to you? If you could only have one, which one would it be?" Keep doing this until you have got the top eight values, and have ranked them from one to eight. Then you do this for all the areas listed above, so you find all the values, and you rank them according to their importance. Or at the very least find your values in the area of your life in which your biggest problem lies.

Step 2: Classifying values as positive or negative
Your Angel Coach now asks, "Why is X value important to you?" Your answer will give you a good indication of whether the value is associated with positive or negative energy.

After this you need to find out if this particular value is a positive or negative value. For example, say someone has love as a value and they are asked, "Why is love important to you?" Perhaps Person A says love is important to them because they never felt love as a child. They have a negative representation of love – of not getting it as a child – and there's a good chance that they might have some strong Negative Emotions and thoughts associated with their past experiences of love.

Then they are asked, "How much negative or positive energy do you have associated with this on a scale from 100 per cent negative to 100 per cent positive? If you were to place yourself on this scale [see page117], where would you place yourself?"

They may say it is 90 per cent negative. I now know that they have many Negative Emotions and deep wounds in relation to love and as a coach I need to find the structure of these wounds (Problem Strategies, Limiting Beliefs, Negative Emotions, Parts Conflicts) and facilitate my client's healing. Doing that will change their value of love and after the full intervention, when we re-elicit their values and they again say "love", if I have done my job well they will be left with the value of love being filled with 100 per cent Positive Energy (Positive Thoughts and Emotions), helping them to move toward creating love in their lives.

Person B might say that love is important to them because it just "is". Love is what makes the world go round; what makes it meaningful. When asked how much positive or negative energy they feel in association with this they might say it is 100 per cent positive. I now know that this person has no issues in relation to love.

Keep doing this with all your values and then keep this list, because after you have done the intervention in Part 5 (see pages 188–220), you will compare this first list of values with your new list.

What to watch out for

Remember to watch out for wanting something to appear better than it actually is. An example might be someone who has relationship issues where she feels that she and her partner are arguing all the time, and who also has a relationship value of acceptance. If I ask her where on the scale acceptance is and she says it is 90 per cent toward, but I calibrate that this does not add up with what she has told me earlier, I can then ask, "How much acceptance do you experience in your relationship now?" She might then reply, "Not much at all." I then ask, "OK, so where is acceptance then on this scale, as your relationship is now?"

Prime Concerns

A Prime Concern is the deepest part of the linguistic deep structure of meaning. Anything below a Prime Concern is not "speakable", or it ends up in vague feelings. A Prime Concern will be semantically packed, which means it is accompanied by expressive tonality and physiology, and may also carry many meanings. They are a universal experience, in that most of us have a Prime Concern. The following exercise is a quick way of finding your deepest problems, your deepest Prime Concern, and this can be in words, feelings, Limiting Beliefs and even Parts Conflicts.

The following questions will help to identify your Prime Concerns:

"Best and worst at" elicitation

1. What are you best at? Starting things? Changing things (or continuing with things, keeping them going)? Stopping things (completing things)?
2. What are you worst at? Starting things? Changing things (continuing/ keeping them going)? Stopping things (completing things)?
3. So what is it that you are not being/doing/having that you want to be/do/have?

If you have answered that you are worst at starting things – then ask yourself, "So what am I not being that I want to be?"

If you are worst at changing things or keeping them going, ask yourself, "So what am I not doing that I want to do?"

If you are worst at stopping or completing things, ask yourself, "So what am I not having that I want to have?"

Starting = Being
Changing = Doing
Stopping = Having

Now we will move on to more Prime Concern elicitation. This one is the Ecstatic State elicitation. Here we are not really looking for the ecstatic state, but the non-mirror image reverse (which means opposite in non-NLP language).

Ecstatic State elicitation

Question 1 Can you remember a time when you were totally "ecstatic" (so totally enthusiastic, happy and filled with positive feelings)? A specific time? Good, so go back to that time now, float inside your body, see what you saw, feel what you felt, hear what you heard and notice what you noticed.

Question 2 As you remember that time (when you were totally ecstatic), what was present in that state that is usually not present?

Question 3 What was missing that is usually present in your normal waking state?

Write down your answers, word for word. Always write everything down exactly as you say it, because otherwise you will change the meaning these words hold for your Unconscious Mind. The answers you give to Questions 2 and 3 will give you a level of words that are either Prime Concerns or leading to a Prime Concern.

Hot on the trail

Can you remember an occasion when you were "hot on the trail", really going for something full steam ahead, but you didn't get it?

1. Why didn't you get it?
2. What stopped you?
3. How did the situation appear to you?
4. What did you say to yourself?
5. What purpose was served by the block?
6. What purpose was served by the thing you were "hot on the trail" for?

How do you release a Prime Concern?

You can release a Prime Concern with the Higher-Self Healing Process in Part 5 (see pages 195–9). You can also release it with the non-mirror image reverse inductive language patterns (see Part 3, pages 162–4). So remember which ones were your own Prime Concerns and then make sure you release them later on.

The Power of Linguistics

NLP is famous for its sophisticated linguistics and you will now learn truly how to become a magician with your words. The way we use linguistics in NLP is perhaps not grammatically correct — we are using them to affect someone's internal representation, to challenge the boundaries of a problem, to get the person to notice something they might not have yet noticed, and also to confuse the Conscious Mind so that we can have direct communication with the Unconscious Mind. Hence, some of the linguistics may not make sense to you and that is OK, because confusion always precedes enlightenment. So just allow yourself to relax, trust your Unconscious Mind that it can learn anything – *anything*. It is an amazing source of wisdom and intelligence. After all, it is keeping you alive, it draws breath into your lungs and then expels it again, it causes your heart to beat and it causes your body to digest your food for you. All you have to do is to be willing to give it the time, space and energy that it needs and your Unconscious Mind will learn these linguistics instantaneously, at the speed of lightning, or maybe even quicker than that.

Chapter 8
The Art of Language
in NLP

NLP uses a range of highly sophisticated linguistic patterns. Before we examine the various linguistic patterns, let us first cover some basics, in the form of linguistic presuppositions. These are just to help you to better understand the linguistic patterns later on.

The Foundation Level of NLP Linguistics

Linguistic presuppositions

1. **Existence** – listen for nouns (anything you can put "a", "an" or "one" in front of): "a table", "a house", "an emotion", "one love", "one insight", "one learning", "one understanding".
2. **Possibility/necessity** – listen for modal operators of possibility/ impossibility ("can", "can't", "will", "won't", "may", "may not", "possible", "impossible") and necessity ("should", "shouldn't", "must", "must not", "have to", "need to", "it is necessary"). For example, "I have to do this", "You must learn this", "It is possible to understand this."
3. **Cause and effect** – listen for "makes" and "if ... then", "because". For example, "Learning this now makes it easier for you to heal your life." "*If* you do this now, *then* you can enjoy your lunch later." "I meditate every morning *because* I want to feel happy and balanced throughout the day."
4. **Complex equivalence** – listen for "is", "are", "means". For example, "Learning this is easy and fun", "Healing *means* you are changing."
5. **Awareness** – listen for verbs relating to senses – so see, hear, smell, taste, feel ("notice", "look", "view") and awareness. For example, "Notice how much you have learnt already."

6. **Time** – listen for verb tense, as well as "stop", "now" and "yet". For example, "Practising this now prepares you for healing yourself later. We *have done* this." (Verb tense here tells you that it has happened previously.)

7. **Adverb/adjective** – listen for words adding detail (descriptions) to verbs and nouns. When you describe details of a verb (a verb is something you do, so you can put "to" in front of it; "to sing", "to write", "to learn") you get an adverb. For example "Let your Unconscious Mind guide you to learn this *easily* and *effortlessly* now" (describes how you learn). When you describe/add details to a noun you get an adjective. For example, "Learning this allows you to heal your *amazing* life" (describes how your life is).

8. **Exclusive and inclusive "or"** – listen for "or". Exclusive "or" is like an exclusive club: whichever "or" you choose you will end up with the same result. An example of exclusive "or" is the question, "Do you want to learn this now or in five minutes?". An example of inclusive "or" is the question, "Do you want to learn presuppositions now or the Meta Model?" – this includes a choice of whether you want to learn presuppositions or the Meta Model.

9. **Ordinal** – listen for lists, numbers, orders and sequences, such as "first", "last", "next". For example, "*First* we learn about presuppositions, *next* we learn about the Meta Model."

The Meta Model

Now it is time to go fishing! In NLP we do a lot of fishing, enabling us to find the lynchpin of the structure of the problem that someone has. Some of your fishing tools are the Meta Model questions.

The Meta Model was created as a result of Bandler and Grinder modelling the language patterns of Virginia Satir, one of the best family therapists there has ever been. Virginia had an ability to ask questions of people to really get to the root of the problem. Bandler and Grinder used their modelling technique to enable other people to ask the same kinds of questions and get the same kinds of results – this is called the "Meta Model".

Distortion, generalization and deletion

Bandler and Grinder noticed that when people talk they naturally go through three processes with their language, as a result of inner screening systems. These three processes Bandler and Grinder named "distortion", "generalization" and "deletion".

We *distort* the information by making it fit our own internal model of the world, rather than what is actually happening. We *generalize* the information when we make assumptions about other people based on previous experiences. We *delete* information when we are not telling the whole story.

Surface structure

In NLP terms the words that come out of somebody's mouth are called the "surface structure", so you can say that the words are what you can see on the surface or even above it (imagine that the surface is like the surface of the ocean). However, this surface structure is generated from the deep structure, the one that is deep within somebody's Unconscious Mind, and before it reaches the surface structure it goes through various distortions, deletions and generalizations. Using our Meta Model questions we are able to find the material that has been distorted, generalized and deleted. This enables us to start catching that monster fish that is truly the one creating problems, both beneath the surface and above it. The person may be aware that she has a problem and she might even have an idea what that problem is caused by, but she also knows instinctively that the real problem lies deeper than that – she can feel the presence of that monster fish – she just does not know the structure of it yet. This is what you, as a coach, are fishing for – finding the structure of this monster fish. It is important to get the deep structure, because the deeper you go, the deeper the healing will be. We could work with the surface structure and we would achieve some results, but the deep structure of the problem would still be there, so we would then just keep generating other examples of the same problem. So we want to use Meta Model questions to find what the problem really is about, within the deep structure.

The Meta Model questions enable us to dig down, so we are working with the deep structure. They help us to chunk down, to move from the abstract, global thinking into the concrete, specific details in this scenario; into the specific details of the structure of the problem; into the thought patterns lying underneath.

Meta Model Distortions – Changing meanings ("How?")

1. **Mind-reading** (knowing someone's internal state).
   For example: "She does not like me."
   Meta Question: "How do you know she doesn't like you?"
   Meta Question: "What's your evidence for that?"
2. **Lost performative** (value judgment where the person doing the judging is left out). For example: "It's bad to argue with your parents."
   Meta Question: "Who says it's bad?" Effect: recovers source of belief.
   Meta Question: "How do you know it is bad?"
   Meta Question: "According to whom?"
3. **Cause and effect** (where the cause is, if wrongly put outside of self).
   For example: "He makes me mad."
   Meta Question: "How does what he is doing cause you to choose to feel mad?"
   Meta Question: "How specifically?"
4. **Complex equivalence** (=) (two experiences interpreted as synonymous).
   For example: "Her yelling at me means she doesn't like me."
   Meta Question: "How does her yelling at you mean she does not like you?"
   Meta Question: "Have you ever yelled at someone you like?"

Meta Model Generalizations – Expanding limits ("What?")

1. **Universal quantifiers** (all, every, never, everyone, no one, etc.).
   For example: "He never talks to me" or "All men are stupid."
   Meta Question: "Never? All men?"
   Meta Question: "What would happen if he did talk to you?"
2. **Modal operators**
   a) Modal operators of necessity (required) – should, shouldn't, must, must not, have to, need to, it is necessary.
   For example: "I have to work hard."

Meta Question: "What would happen if you didn't?"
Meta Question: "What wouldn't happen if you didn't?" (Don't worry if this question does not make sense. It won't unless you have a problem, and then when someone asks you this question you find that you can suddenly answer it!)
Meta Question: "Or?"
b) Modal operators of possibility (or impossibility) – can, can't, will, won't, may, may not, possible, impossible.
For example: "I can't stop smoking."
Meta Question: "What prevents you?" Effect: recovers causes
Meta Question: "What would happen if you did?"
Meta Question: "What would happen if you didn't?"

Meta Model Deletions – Gathering information

1. **Nominalizations** (process words, verbs that have been turned into nouns, such as to communicate (verb)/communication (noun).
   For example: "We have a problem with our communication."
   Meta Question: "How would you like to communicate?" Effect: turns it back into a process.
   Meta Question: "Who is not communicating what to whom?"

2. **Unspecified verbs**
   For example: "He annoys me."
   Meta Question: "How specifically does he annoy you?"

3. **Comparative deletions** (good, better, worst, more, less, least)
   For example: "She is a better person."
   Meta Question: "Compared to what/who?"
   Meta Question: "Better than who?"

Making the Meta Model work

1. Building rapport (see pages 39–47).
2. Using softening frames, such as, "I'm wondering", "I'm curious", "That's interesting".
3. Questioning clients' statements – check a distortion, generalization or deletion, and then ask a Meta Model question to help identify the source of the distortion, deletion or generalization.

The Milton Model

Many years ago, I felt something stirring inside me. At first I did not know what it was, but slowly and steadily this inner feeling became stronger. Something within me wanted me to change. I don't know if you have ever felt this, you probably have. Just as you are sitting reading this, thinking many thoughts, feeling many feelings deep inside, I am sure you, too, at times have felt something within you changing, evolving, wanting you to become more and more who you truly are. I remember I felt as if I had outgrown my old outside self, as if I had a cocoon around me and something beautiful wanted to come out, to be free, so that I could be, do and have everything I was meant to be, do and have. And I heard this inner voice saying to me:

"I know you are curious and it is good to be curious, because it allows you to seek solutions and that means you are learning, healing, growing and changing on many levels now, and you can learn, grow, heal and change in many ways, creating new learnings, insights and integrations, just as you have now, haven't you? People can, you know, learn in many ways and this is a better way of doing it, as you sit here, listening to me, thinking many thoughts. Your Unconscious Mind can make all the integrations it needs for learning instantaneously or maybe even quicker than that. Do you realize this is something you can do? Speaking to you as a wise person, who knows that learning, growing, healing and changing can be easy and fun, allowing you to become everything you are meant to be."

So what did I just do? I introduced you to the Milton Model, where we use artfully vague linguistics in order to induce trance.

What is the Milton Model?

The Milton Model was created by Bandler and Grinder, modelling the language patterns of Milton Erickson, enabling you to begin to create the hypnotic language patterns that he used. These patterns are artfully vague, so that when you are using the Milton Model language patterns with someone their Conscious Mind very quickly becomes overloaded, because every single statement you make can have several different meanings. So the person's Conscious Mind starts thinking, "Does it mean this or does it mean that? Could it be this? Could it be that?" While the client's Conscious Mind is busy working that out you fire off another Milton Model Pattern, which very quickly overloads your client's Conscious Mind, and the client then begins to go into a trance.

What can we use the Milton Model for?

We can use it to induce trance; light, medium and deep trance, and also to increase rapport because your language is so artfully vague it allows the other person to fit their Model of the World onto what you are saying, so they think you actually think the same way as them – that is the perception you are creating.

The Milton Model uses the following patterns to allow you to communicate directly with the person's Unconscious Mind:

1. **Mind-reading** – claiming to know the thoughts or feelings of another without specifying how you know what they are thinking or feeling.

   Sample phrases: "I know you know, you know ...", " I know you are wondering ...", "I know you are curious." "I know you are healing ...".

2. **Lost performative** – a statement that makes a judgment but does not specify who made the judgment.

   Sample phrases: "It makes a lot of sense ..." , "And it is good to be curious ..."

3. **Cause and Effect** – a statement that implies that one thing causes another: "... causes ...", If ... then ...", "As you ... then you ...", "While ... then ...", "... makes ..."

   Sample phrases: "And that is because I can see it in your eyes." "Eating fish makes you clever." "Healing this makes you happier."

4. **Complex Equivalence** – where two things are said to be the same, have the same meaning, or happen simultaneously (the verb "to be")

   Sample phrases: "And that means ...", "You are healing ...", "I am learning this now."

5. **Universal quantifiers** – words with universal generalizations and no referential index. Such as: all, never, every, always.

   Sample phrases: "On every level", "All of the time ..."

6. **Modal operators** – words that imply possibility/impossibility or necessity/negative necessity. They tend to form the rules we have in our lives, such as can, will, must, ought, possible, may, may not.
   Sample phrases: "Simply because we have to …", "and you can learn many things …"

7. **Nominalizations** – verbs frozen in time, making them nouns.
   "Create new learnings, integrations, communication, changes …"

8. **Unspecified verbs** – verbs that delete the specifics of how, when and where.
   Sample phrases: "And you can …", "That you have now …"

9. **Tag question** – a closed question added to the end of a statement to displace resistance.
   Sample phrases: "Can't you?", "Haven't you?", "Don't you?"

10. **Lack of referential index** – a statement in which it is not clear specifically who the statement refers to.
    Sample phrases: "People can, you know …", "No one likes to do this …", "Everyone will love this."

11. **Comparative deletions** – (unspecified comparison) – where a comparison is made and it is not specified against what or who the comparison was made.
    Sample phrases: "That's the major difference with healing in this way." "This is a better way of doing it."

12. **Pacing current experience** – undeniably (so the client cannot deny the truth of what you are saying) describing the client's internal and external experience.
    Sample phrase: "And as you sit there, looking at the book, reading these words etc."

13. **Double binds** – where an illusion of choice is created, but no matter which choice is taken the outcome is the same.
    Sample phrases: "You're unconscious … can make the integrations it needs instantaneously or maybe even quicker than that."

14. **Conversational postulate** – a closed question that creates an internal representation of something you want the client to do. It allows the client to choose to respond, or not, and avoids authoritarianism.
    Sample phrase: "Do you realize this is something you can do?"

15. **Extended quotes** – where it is not possible to discern where one quote leaves off and the next one begins.

    Sample phrases: "I remember being at a seminar and John Grinder mentioned that he had worked with Milton and one of his clients had said …"

16. **Selectional restriction violation** – implying an object or animal can have human responses.

    Sample phrases: "His budget said he had to change in one session …", "You and your chair can go into a deep trance together now."

17. **Ambiguities**

    a) Phonological – where two words sound the same but have different meanings:

    here/hear
    right/rite/write/wright
    there/their/they're
    knows/nose
    pear/pair/pare
    bow/bough

    b) Syntactic – where the function (syntactic) of the word cannot be immediately determined from the context.

    Sample phrases: "They are visiting relatives",

    "They are healing healers".

    (Are "visiting" and "healing" being used as verbs or as adjectives?)

    c) Scope – where it cannot be determined to which portion of a sentence a word applies.

    Sample phrases: "Speaking to you as a wise person …" (Who is the wise person? The person speaking, or the person listening?), "The charming men and women …" (Does "charming" apply to men and women or just men?)

    d) Punctuation – run-on sentences, by using the same word that ends a sentence to begin the next sentence.

    Sample phrases: "It's time to look at your *watch how quickly you change*", "It is easy to learn *linguistics is fun*"

    e) Pause at improper places – The sentence is left unfinished.

    Sample phrases: "I know that you are wondering …" You can …"

18. **Utilization** – you use anything that is happening or is being said, by mentioning it. Because it is actually happening, so is undeniably true, it helps to increase rapport, trust and therefore also trance.

Client says, "I don't understand."

Response: "That's right, you don't understand yet and that's because we haven't done the process that will allow you to totally understand this, and we are just about to do that now ..."

Or, "That's right, you don't understand and that's because you haven't asked the one question that will let you completely understand it all now."

Or another example happened during one of our trainings, when one coach (Rob Purfield, a brilliant NLP Trainer) was working with a student who was easily disturbed by outside noise, so had problems relaxing and following the exercise. It was a hot day, so the windows and doors were open. They could hear the toilet next door flushing, doors closing and opening and the kids playing outside.

Rob said: "Every time you hear a door opening, it is as if you are opening a door into an aspect of your Unconscious Mind, allowing you to change and heal at a very deep level, and every time the door closes, it is as though you are closing the door to an old chapter in your life, allowing you to move on into a positive future. Whenever you hear the toilet flushing, it is as though you are flushing away all that old stuff you are now ready to let go of, while listening to the delightful laughter of your inner child playing freely and happily, ready to enjoy a happy, delightful life."

Every time the door opened or closed or the toilet flushed or the laughter from the kids outside became even stronger, the student used this, with the result that he relaxed and went into a deep trance.

19. **Metaphor** – creating a story for the client's Unconscious Mind to map into resources.

Putting it all together

I know you are curious and it's good to be inquisitive, because it allows you to seek solutions and that means you are growing, learning, healing and changing all the time. Notice how much you are changing on every level now and you can learn and grow in many ways, creating new learnings, insights and integrations, just as you have now, haven't you? People can heal in many ways and this is a better way of doing it, as you sit here, reading these words, thinking many thoughts. Your Unconscious Mind can make all the integrations it needs instantaneously – or maybe even quicker than that. Do you realize this is something you can do? I remember being at a seminar when someone said, "Your Unconscious Mind is very wise", and you and your Unconscious Mind are learning many things together during your life, creating miracles and magic, and your Unconscious Mind knows that healing, growing and changing can be easy and fun.

The difference between the Milton Model and the Meta Model

Milton Model

- Uses vague language to create rapport and induce trance.
- Moves from surface structure to deep structure by enabling the client to focus more internally.
- Aims to access unconscious resources.

Meta Model

- Uses very specific language.
- Aims to bring unconscious patterns, beliefs and thoughts into conscious awareness.

Language frames

Agreement frame

An agreement frame is a way of using language as a frame of respectful agreement when differing opinions are present in a conversation. Use words such as "I appreciate", "and", "I agree", "I respect", "because".

Avoid, "I understand" and "but". When you say, "I understand", the other person may feel, "Well how can you? You are not me!" Saying "but" immediately suggests you don't agree with them, so it negates what you have just said.

"What would happen if you could" frame?

Framing can move people who feel they are stuck and direct them to what they thought they couldn't do. When a person is stuck and says they can't do something, ask, "What would happen if you could?"

"For what purpose?" frame

This kind of framing helps someone to become unstuck by letting them see the bigger picture. Ask, "For what purpose?"

Reframes

Reframes are useful ways of shifting someone's perception. For example, different behaviours have different meanings in different contexts. In the English-speaking world you are taught from a young age the importance of saying "please". In Swedish we do not have a word for "please"; instead we use "thank you". So when we have dinner with someone who has English as their native language, and before we know English well, we may ask a question such as, "Can you pass me the vegetables?"

To a native English speaker that sends shivers down the spine, and inside you are probably screaming, "Please!", because that's the way you were taught to ask for something ever since you were small. Now the Swedish person has no idea that not saying "please" is considered rude, and after you have passed them the vegetables, they say, "Thank you", and that is their way of being polite. It is the same behaviour, but for the English-speaking person it is considered rude and for the Swedish person it is considered polite.

When my daughter was three years old she had tantrums very easily, which would be considered pretty normal – after all, she was only a toddler. Now if I displayed the same behaviour – screaming, throwing myself back and forth, with froth coming out of my mouth, turning blue (because I was so busy screaming that I forgot to breathe), then people would either think I was having a fit or that I belonged in a mental institution. Same behaviour – different contexts.

Reframes are highly useful linguistics to enable someone to shift their thinking, to literally help them to expand their perception, so they are able to "try on" different frames of thinking. It is a useful tool to have in any circumstance in life – with your children, partner, parents, colleagues, neighbours, or with anyone.

The easiest way of doing reframes is actually to not think – instead just trust your Unconscious Mind to say something that would help your client shift their thinking in such a way that a deep healing can take place. You do this naturally with your friends and family, so just use your natural healing ability, which is within your heart. Stop trying, stop thinking and instead just connect with your heart and fully be there for the other person. Then deliver your reframe.

I will now go through some more formal ways of creating reframes and I want you to remember the advice above. The formal ways appeal to the logical Conscious Mind – however it is the Unconscious Mind that is the true genius in delivering reframes. So trust it!

Context reframes

We use a context reframe with a problem that is expressed as a Comparative Deletion; "I'm too …", "He's too …", "They are too …", "It's too …". Also after comparative adjectives and adverbs, which generally finish with … "-er" (such as "This is a better way of doing this").

For example, a woman of 37 says, "I am too old to be a parent."

Reframe: "Imagine how much wisdom and patience you have learnt over the years, which you can then pass on to your children."

For example, "It is too late for me to change now. I have already damaged my children." (This is something I often hear from parents.)

Reframe: "Can you imagine if your parents had changed when you were the age your children are now? How would that have affected you if your parents had allowed themselves to be happy, fulfilled and embracing life? How would that have benefited you?"

When a problem comes along that is expressed like this you think of a different context in which the problem behaviour might have a different meaning.

Ask yourself: "Where would this behaviour be useful (have value)?

In which context would this behaviour be useful?"

When we deliver that to the client, it changes their Internal Representation and therefore changes their state and their behaviour.

Meaning reframe

We use meaning reframes when the problem is expressed as a Complex Equivalence or Cause and Effect. Whenever X, I respond Y. A causes B.

What we are going to do here is keep the problem the same internally, in the same context, but we want to change the meaning of it.

There are a number of ways of doing this.

- We could ask ourselves what else could X mean?
- Or we could think of an opposite frame.

Or we could ask ourselves:

- What hasn't this person noticed in this context, which if they did, would change the meaning?
- What other positive value or meaning could this have?

For example, my elder daughter, who is blessed with lovely long, slim legs, once said to me, when she was seven years old, "Mummy, I don't like my legs, because they are too skinny and too long."

So I took her out for a walk with our dog and then we started running and we had great fun. Then I delivered my reframe, "Isn't it great, Erika, that you have such long legs so that you can run so fast! Your legs are incredible, you know. They allow you to do so much fun stuff in life, such as running, climbing, swimming and cycling. Aren't you happy you have such great long, slim legs?" And from that moment to this she has never had a bad word to say about her legs!

Another example: "I don't want to forgive her because she has hurt me so much."

Reframe: "How much energy do you waste by holding on to this old hurt? Imagine how much lighter, freer and more energized you will feel when you forgive her? Did you know that forgiveness is the most selfish act we can carry out, because it frees us from the past? So be really, really selfish and forgive her, so that you are able to move on with your life, living it to the full."

Another example: A client was very angry with her ex-husband, because he had left her to be with another woman. She had been angry with him for over 10 years and this was now affecting her new marriage quite badly, so she came to see me. During the case history it was revealed that my client had, in fact, also been unfaithful to her ex-husband in the early years of their marriage. Her ex-husband knew about the affair, since she was going to leave him, but then her lover decided he did not want to be with her, so she went back to her husband instead – who took her back!

My client said, "I can't let go of my anger toward my ex-husband, because he left me. I am so angry with him for leaving me and that means I can't enjoy my life now."

Reframe: "Wouldn't it be easier to get on with your life and be happy if you let your anger go?"

Reframe: "How do you think your husband felt when you had the affair early in your marriage?" (You need lots of rapport to do this one. In this case, it was the reframe that shifted the whole problem, because it allowed her to see that, in fact, she had had a role to play in her husband eventually leaving her. Realizing this, she could easily let go of her anger and blame and it stopped her from seeing herself as a victim).

Reframe with the highest intention

The premise is that all behaviour has a positive intention, therefore a problem is a problem because it is in conflict with the highest intention of the behaviour. We here use chunking-up questions, such as: For what purpose? What is the highest intention?

For example, say we do not want to let go of sadness. As we ask, "For what purpose?" We might then get the answer, "Protection." We then ask, "For what purpose?" The answer is now, "Safety." For what purpose? "Happiness."

We have now found a conflict between sadness and happiness, as they are the opposite to each other. Our reframe here could then be: "So wouldn't it be easier to be happy if you let the sadness go?"

Chapter 9
Becoming a Magician with Your Words

Advanced Presuppositions

Now we are going to cover Advanced Presuppositions, which are advanced linguistic patterns. The key here is to just look at the structure of the sentences and then come up with your own example. We use these types of linguistic patterns all the time (well, perhaps not always, unless you are already trained in NLP), so they are easier when you just do them, instead of trying to consciously understand them by applying logic and reason. So just get on with it and *do* them!

Existence [noun]: The question here is: Are you sure?
   Evidence challenge with **not + time**
   Example: "I have depression."
   Response: "When are you sure it is not there?"

   Example: "I have stress in my life."
   Response: "When are you sure it is not there?"

Possibility: If it is a modal operator of impossibility, remember it is the process of "I can do X of not". For example, "It is impossible for me to change", means it is the process of not being able to do the changing.
   So the question here can be: "How can you not … change?" Or: "How can you choose … to not change?"
   Example: "I can't stop shouting at the kids."
   Response: "How can you not … stop shouting?"

   Example: "It is impossible for me to relax."
   Response: "What would your life be like if you could?"

If it is a modal operator of necessity, it is often useful to chain it to a modal operator of possibility, such as connecting, "I must change this now" to, "I know you feel you must change this now, but how would it be if you were to consider that you can indeed change even more if you were to ease the pressure on yourself and give yourself more time?" (We will cover chaining of modal operators on pages 143–6.)

Complex Equivalence: Take the opposite, pace it to the limit (so you take it as far out to the boundary as you can), and use a counter example with a Referential Index switch (you do this in the same way as a Perceptual Position switch, see pages 59–63) to the solution.

Example: "You never giving me flowers means you don't love me."
Response: "How much love will the flowers need to give before you know I do?"
Response: "Imagine how our love will blossom when you trust that I do."

Example: "Not knowing why I am sad means I cannot heal."
Response: "How much more healing will it be for your sadness when you just know you can?"
Response: "How much more do you need to know before you realize you already have everything within you for your healing?"

Cause and Effect: Switch positions, exaggerate the effect, switch Referential Index and do a "not" on the cause.

Example: "I can't do this, because I don't understand it."
Response: "How much more totally understanding will it be when you do."

Example: "I can't let this anger go, because my parents never loved me."
Response: "How much more loving will you feel inside when you let the anger go?"

Example: "I can't tell my husband how I feel about his new job, because he may not love me then."
Response: "How fantastic will he feel when you trust him enough to let him show you his love?"

Response: "How totally unloved do you think he feels when he realizes you have not shared your innermost feelings with him?"

Time: Since time is a nominalization (a verb that has been frozen in time, by making it a noun), you can use time as a decision destroyer (so you help to use the linguistics of time to destroy Limiting Beliefs and Decisions).

Example: "Before I can love him, I must trust him."
Response: "How much more loving will he be when you do trust him?
Response: "How much more trusting will you be in yourself when you do?"

Example: "Before I can let this depression go, I must have a future to look forward to."
Response: "How much greater will your future be, when you let your depression go?"

Adjective/adverb: Comparative deletions (see page 131); same behaviour, different context.

Example: "My teenage daughter is too argumentative."
Response: "Isn't it fantastic that she is learning to speak her mind and stand up for herself?"

Inclusive/exclusive "or":
Example: "I can't decide whether I should commit to her or not."
Response: "How will you ever be able to commit to anything if you do not make up your mind and just decide?"

Example: "I can't decide whether I should focus on my spiritual development or not."
Response: "So if you don't allow yourself to get to know your soul, how will you be able to find out what you want to create in life?"

Ordinal: Reverse the order and apply one on top of the other.
Example: "I need to know why I am depressed before I can allow myself to be happy."
Response: "Why don't you allow yourself to be happy while you find out?"

Meta Model III

Directed questioning for a specific result

Now we are going to cover Meta Model III questioning techniques, which are sophisticated tools to facilitate deep change in someone. These techniques are very useful when working with yourself or with others. Think of a problem you have and then run it through these questions focusing on the problem.

Start

1. "What's the problem?"
2. "How do you know it is a problem?"
3. "When did you decide that it was a problem?" (Cause)
4. "What other positive choices could you have made to solve this problem now?" (This is a "flip-over" question, helping to "flip" the problem over from being viewed from a problem angle to being viewed from the solution angle.)
5. "How is that different from how you were?"
6. "How do you know that now?"

During the first three questions you are taken deeper into the problem and you also get to the cause. The fourth question is a flip-over question and you then are able to flip the problem over to the solution. The last two questions are deepening solution questions.

How did it feel to have a problem and run it through the questions like that? Quite interesting isn't it, how you linguistically can start to find the solutions? This is what you do in Break-Through Healing sessions too. The beginning of the session is when all the detective work is done and you start to diagnose the structure of the problem. You also loosen it up so much that it is already on the move and halfway through the door before you even start with the intervention.

Let us do another example. So think of another problem and run it through another set of Meta Model III questions:

1. "So what is going on?"
2. "How do you do that?"

3. "When don't you do it?"
4. "What are the Positive Learnings here so you are able to solve this now?" (Flip-over)
5. "How will you be different when you have solved it?"
6. "In how many ways will your life be enriched when you have made this change to solve that old problem?"

Now come up with your own Meta Model III questions. With the first three go deeper and deeper into the problem to find the strategy and cause. Then you have a flip-over question and then you find the solution questions, which will also help to reassure you that you have indeed found the solution. You can have as few as six to eight questions if you want. Identify your flip-over question.

Linguistic submodalities

Have you ever had the experience of talking to someone who knows about NLP and just by talking to her, you start to feel better. Say, for example, you feel you just can't do something and your NLP friend then says, "I know you feel you can't do this, but how would it be if you were to allow yourself to consider the possibility that perhaps you can ... do this now."

Your mind starts going round and round in circles and before you know it you are doing exactly the thing that you previously felt you couldn't.

We are going to cover briefly how you can chain (link together) modal operators.

Let us first classify the modal operators again:

1) **Negative necessity** – words such as "must not", "ought not", "shouldn't", "don't have to", "doesn't allow to", "supposed not to", "not necessarily".
2) **Improbability** – words such as "couldn't", "might not", "wouldn't", "had better not", "may not", "don't dare to", "don't wish to", "don't let".
3) **Impossibility** – words such as "am not", "can't", "try not", "unable to", "won't", "don't intend to", "impossible", "don't decide".
4) **Necessity** – words such as "allow", "got to", "must", "necessary", "ought to", "should", "supposed to", "have to", "it's time to".

5) **Probability** – words such as "could", "dare to", "had better", "prefer", "pretend", "wish", "may", "let", "deserve", "might".
6) **Possibility** – words such as "could", "might", "prefer", "wish", "pretend", "would", "had better", "dare to", "may", "possible", "will", "can".

You probably realize that the words within Probability and Possibility are similar, because they both work within a similar mode – both imply "probability" and "possibility", which are similar in themselves.

"Chaining" modal operators means that you detect the negative modal operators someone is using and you then "chain" these negative modal operators until you end up with a modal operator of probability or possibility. This will change your client's Internal Representation, from a negative Internal Representation to a positive Internal Representation, just by using language structure.

For example, someone says, "I really don't want to let go of my anger toward my … [in-law, spouse, parent, sibling]. It is too deep-seated."

You say, "I know you don't want to let go of your anger. I know you don't have to consider the possibility that perhaps you could, just for a moment at least, give yourself the gift of deserving to be free from this anger. How much better would you feel inside if you did … let go of that old anger now? Could you then perhaps realize that this is something you can do?"

Someone says, "I can't change."

You say, "I know you think you can't change and some people feel it might even be impossible to change or that it is too late to change, and maybe they shouldn't have to think that … they can change, because we all change all the time. As you are sitting here now you are a different person from the person you were five years ago, or one year ago, or even one month ago, because change happens all the time, in the same way that the cells inside your body change constantly, you also change inside. You cannot not change; change is part of life and perhaps this is a better way of doing it, just allowing change to happen, and perhaps you can now recognize that you can indeed change?"

To help you chain modal operators look at the table opposite.

1. Negative necessity
Not necessary
Need not
Supposed not to
It's not time
Must not
Doesn't allow to
Ought not
Don't have to
Shouldn't
Got to not

2. Improbability
Had better not
Couldn't
Might not
Don't dare to
Don't prefer
Don't wish
Don't deserve
Wouldn't
Don't let
Don't pretend

3. Impossibility
Unable to
Can't
Won't
Am not
Try not
Don't intend to
Don't choose to
Doesn't permit
Don't decide
Impossible

4. Necessity
Necessary
Ought to
Have to
It's time
Must
Allow
Got to
Need to
Should
Supposed to

5. Probability
Wish
Prefer
Deserve
Had better
Dare to
Could
Might
Would
Let
Pretend

6. Possibility
Am
Can
Permit
Choose to
Try
Intend to
Possible
Will
Decide
Able to

To chain modal operators go round clockwise. You start at 3, go up to 2, 1, 4, 5 and finish at 6. Move clockwise and end up in Group 6 (Possibility) or Group 5 (Probability).

Let me give you an example, and I will use the words in the box on the previous page, so we have "Can't" (Group 3), "Don't have to" (Group 1), "It's time" (Group 4), "Pretend" (Group 5) and "Can" (Group 6).

Example: "I can't learn how to do this."

Response: "I know you feel you can't learn how to do this, and perhaps you don't have to learn this now, but how would it be if you imagined it now was time to at least choose to pretend that indeed you can … learn this now."

Linguistic submodalities for space

You know that our words affect our Internal Representation, because every word will mean something different and we store our meanings in different submodalities. We also have different submodalities, which affect our perception of space. Words that affect our Internal Representation of space are, for example: "across", "after", "alongside", "apart from", "at", "before", "behind", "beside", "between", "beyond", "down", "from above", "from below", "in", "including", "in front of", "in place of", "inside", "into", "off", "on", "onto", "out of", "outside", "over", "relative to", "sort of", "through", "toward", "under", "up" and "with", as well as "within" and "without".

You also have some spatial predicates that affect whether the Internal Representation is associated or disassociated, such as "here – there", "this – that".

We use linguistic submodalities constantly – such as: "Move that problem to one side now", "Beyond the horizon lies your dreams", "I am always here beside you", "Let the light go before you and guide you on your path, "From above came the answers" and so on.

Let me give you examples of using linguistic submodalities on space:

"Please bring up your old problem in your mind now. As you think about this old problem, what is the solution that lies within it, because you know, don't you, that every problem contains its own solution. So allow your mind's inner eye now to see and feel this solution within your old problem. Just notice what it is and then allow this solution to rise up over your old problem, allowing you to see, feel and notice it clearly."

"How would it be if you just moved that old problem to the side, so that your solution can be revealed, which is lying behind it?"

"How about if you just cut through that old fear and instead allowed all your inner resources to come up in place of that old fear?"

Using words to presuppose permanence
(of positive change or anything else that is positive)

Here are some examples of words that presuppose permanence:

"Lasting", "enduring", "persisting", "persistent", "long-standing", "forever and ever", "perpetual", "always", "goes on and on", "stable", "eternal", "long-lasting", "constant".

So you can use these words to help someone have an Internal Representation of a permanent change, by saying things such as, "So allow these great feelings inside now to go on forever and ever, just allow it to go on and on, into eternity, as a constant, lasting, enduring great feeling. Just go out into the future now and fill it with these great feelings, and then take them all the way out into eternity, filling your future with ... [whatever positive emotions they have given you previously, such as light, love, compassion or understanding]." (Be sure to use the person's exact words for their recourses, rather than what you think they should have been.)

Words that presuppose impermanence

Here are some examples of words that presuppose impermanence:

"Fleeting", "short-term", "in the blink of an eye", "short-lived", "here today gone tomorrow", "temporary", "unstable", "brief", "melt like snow".

You can use the words and phrases to imply the impermanence of your client's problem, such as, "As you think of that fleeting old problem, just know how it can disappear *in the blink of an eye*, be *here today and gone tomorrow*. Just as the snow is really thick and deep during the winter, as you bring in the light and warmth of the sun, the snow just *melts* away, and as you bring in the light of your awareness and the warmth of your love and compassion, your old problem can also just *melt away like snow*."

Remembering	**Forgetting**
Recall	A mind like a sieve
Fix in your mind	Slip one's mind
Bear in mind	Remember to forget
Keep in mind	Think nothing of it
Bring it up in your mind now	Lose your train of thought
Etched upon your brain	Forget to remember
Refresh your mind	Gone with the wind
Bring to the front of your mind now	Put it to the back of your mind
Fix your sight on it	Out of sight, out of mind

Examples of how to use this:

- "Now think of a problem you have, bring it up in your mind now – and your mind is like a sieve sometimes, isn't it? – and you just remember to forget, or is it that you forget to remember, and you sometimes just feel how you lose your train of thought and you think nothing of it, it is as though it has just gone with the wind, as if it has just slipped your mind, it is out of sight, out of mind."
- "Think now of that old problem you have. Bring it into your mind now and as you do so, allow the solution that is present within this problem to pop up into your mind, just allow it to shine its light now onto this old problem, so that the old problem is transformed. What is this solution? Notice what it is. Now allow this solution to be fixed in your mind, fix your sight on it and really etch it upon your brain, so that you can easily recall it at any time when you need it, whenever you need to refresh your mind about the solution, just like you have now, haven't you?"

Going beyond words: a de-identification pattern

No matter what you think you are, you are always more than that. This is a highly useful technique for challenging and transcending boundary conditions with Complex Equivalences, which are language constructions of identification. You can also use this technique on yourself. When I did this during my own Master Practitioner training I ended up going to the point just before my own conception and I could see, hear, feel and experience myself in space, as a spirit, sitting there looking out at my life ahead of me and preparing myself for the journey, thinking, "Oh, my God! What a ride this is going to be!" I knew I had set myself some really tough challenges and I heard a voice saying, "Are you sure you want to do this?" and I answered a fully congruent, "Yes, I am!"

Exercise to do with a partner

First you elicit the identification in the form of a Complex Equivalence. You look for the verb "to be", such as "I am", or the word "means".

1. First you pace and feed back (so you read back the sentence to your client) the Complex Equivalence. "So you are _____ [statement they made]?" This makes them present-state associated, which means they bring up the physiology of the Complex Equivalence into their mind and body.
2. "Is that all you think you are?" (Look for a physiological shift.)
3. "Aren't you more than that?" (There should be agreement.)
4. "What are you that is not _____ [the previous identification]?" You want a verbal answer here, because you need a word to continue the process.
5. "And beyond _____ [word they gave you], is that all you are? Aren't you more than that? You do know that you are more than that, don't you? What are you that is not _____ [the previous identification?" Or you may want to ask if what they gave you was already a positive, "What are you that is even more than _____ ?"

   You keep going with Step 5 until you get the non-mirror image reverse (meaning "opposite" in normal language) of their original statement, such as from "I am bad" to "I am good". They will get to a "beyond word" state, such as I did when I floated back to the point before my own conception.
6. Once you get the non-mirror image reverse, that is, the opposite to the statement they started with, such as from "I am bad" to "I am good", you then ask them, "Is this the place your Unconscious Mind wants you to get to?" If you calibrate a "Yes" from the person's Unconscious Mind, you then ask, "How do you know?" This

anchors the change to the person's reality strategy. If the person's Unconscious Mind says "No", you keep doing Step 5 until you reach the level the person's Unconscious Mind wants to get to.

An example of this is the following:

Person A says, "I am a bad person."

Person B says, "So you are a bad person? Is that all you think you are? Aren't you more than that? What are you that is not a bad person?"

A: "A good person."

B: "And beyond that. Is that all you are? Aren't you more than that? You do know you are more than that, don't you? What are you, that is even more than being a good person?"

A: "I am wonderful."

B: "And beyond that. Is that all you are? Aren't you more than that? You do know you are more than that, don't you? What are you, that is even more than wonderful?"

A: "I am connected with the Divine."

B: "Ask your Unconscious Mind if this is the level you need to get to."

A: "Yes" (but the coach calibrates a "No" signal).

B: "And beyond that. Is that all you are? Aren't you more than that? You do know you are more than that, don't you? What are you, that is even more than being connected with the Divine?"

A: "I am an eternal Spirit filled with love."

B: "Ask your Unconscious Mind if this is the level you need to get to."

A: "Yes" (and the coach calibrates a "Yes" signal, too).

B: "How do you know you are an eternal Spirit filled with love?"

A: "I feel it here [points to heart], and I see purple and white sparkling colours everywhere."

Chapter 10
Advanced Hypnotic NLP Linguistics

Hypnotic patterns of Milton Erickson

Milton Erickson, a great American hypnotherapist and one of the three outstanding therapists Grinder and Bandler modelled when they founded NLP, believed that the Unconscious Mind was always listening, and that whether or not the person was in trance, suggestions could be made that would have a hypnotic influence, as long as those suggestions found some resonance at the unconscious level. You can be aware of this, or you can be completely oblivious that something is happening ... now.

Erickson maintained that trance is a common, everyday occurrence. For example, you can go into a light trance while waiting for the bus, reading a book, listening to music or in the moment just before dropping off to sleep. At such moments people experience the common everyday trance; they tend to gaze off and get that "blank" look.

Erickson maintained that it was not possible to consciously instruct the Unconscious Mind and that authoritarian suggestions were likely to be met with resistance. The Unconscious Mind responds to openings, opportunities, metaphors and contradictions. Effective hypnotic suggestion, then, should be "artfully vague", leaving space for the client to fill in the gaps with their own unconscious understandings – even if they do not consciously grasp what is happening.

We are now going to cover some of the hypnotic language patterns that Erickson used most often.

Direct and indirect suggestions

A direct suggestion appeals directly to the Conscious Mind, which has the opportunity to evaluate the suggestion. For example, "Do this process now." "Let go of your anger now."

An indirect suggestion appeals to the Unconscious Mind and is not evaluated as much (and therefore not resisted as much by the Conscious Mind). For example, "I am wondering if you can do this process now?", "I am wondering if you can let go of your anger now?"

Embedded commands

This is when you have a command embedded in the middle of a conversation, which bypasses the Conscious Mind. In the examples below, the embedded command is the portion of the sentence that is in italics. You can guide it to the Unconscious Mind by marking it out analogically, so by changing your tone of voice or adopting a specific gesture or changing your body posture.

"I am curious to know if you can *heal this now.*"

"I am wondering if you can *let this sadness go now.*"

Truism about sensations

This is when you make something true about sensations and emotions.

"Most people feel really light and happy as they let their problem go."

"Many people feel happy in their hearts as they realize their own inner power and wisdom."

Truism utilizing time

This is when you make something true using time.

"The solution to your problem can reveal itself now … as you are emotionally and mentally ready."

"Sooner or later you will gain all the insights you need for you to heal this now."

Using "not knowing" and "not doing" as a way to bypass Conscious Mind resistance:

"You can heal and not know you are healing, you can breathe and not be aware that you are breathing; your body just does it all by itself."

"You don't have to do anything to learn this."

Compound suggestions

This is when you use several suggestions to help deepen trance.

Associations: "With every breath you take you can let your body and mind heal even more deeply."

Opposites: "The more you choose to live your life from a place of love, compassion and light, the less attracted you will be to reacting from a place of anger, fear and negativity."

"Yes" set (meaning the client will answer "Yes" internally): "You want to heal, you want to feel better about yourself and your life and you are ready now to let this problem go. Let's start our coaching session now." (What you have done here is intuited that they have repeated an internal "Yes", so that when you then suggest starting the coaching session they tend to say "Yes" to that, too.)

Negative-tag question: "You can heal, can't you?" or "You can learn this now, can't you?"

Negative-until: "You don't have to change until you are ready to heal." "You don't have to learn this until you are ready to grow."

Covering all possibilities of responses

"Soon you will find you are thinking and behaving in a new way, perhaps in a few weeks, months or years, you will look back at today and think, 'Wow, I have learnt so much; I have changed so much since then.'"

Questions to facilitate possibilities of new responses

To facilitate internal change

"How can you best heal and evolve your Inner Self? Will it be because you are learning how to let go of inner pain, by learning how to shine the light of your awareness into the deepest part of your mind and in this way release the essence, the love that is there?"

To focus attention

"Did you experience your meditation state as similar to your normal waking state or different from your normal waking state?"

Open-ended suggestions

"You don't always know how much you are changing and growing and it is not right for me to tell you to change this or change that. Let yourself change now in whatever way you choose, in whichever way you want to grow and evolve."

Implied directive ("if ... then", "as ... while" statements)

a) "As you take a deep breath in, your Unconscious Mind can make all the integrations it needs, while deeply allowing your Inner Self to heal."
b) "If you ask me another question, then all your answers will be revealed by your own Unconscious Mind."

Double binds

a) "Would you like to change now or in five minutes?"
b) "Would you like to heal this now or later?"
c) "You can make all the healing you need instantaneously or perhaps even quicker than that."
d) "Your deep Inner Self, your Unconscious Mind, knows all the answers that your Conscious Mind does not know, and if your Unconscious Mind knows all the answers, then you probably know more, deep inside, than you think you do."

Metaphors

We are all natural story-tellers and metaphors are fantastic tools for facilitating healing in adults and children alike. As soon as you tell others about your day or your life, you will be telling them a story. In NLP we use these natural stories, these metaphors, as a way of getting our message across, leaving it open for the other person's Unconscious Mind to find their own unique, Positive Learnings from the story. In this way you are not telling the client what the learnings are, you are leaving it open for him/her to make their own connections and conclusions about what the story means. If you use stories from your own life, then it is always best to make sure the story is actually true, as this will have a much greater impact on your audience. They can pick up on the authenticity of the story easily.

The main components to think about when you are creating a metaphor are:

• Decide on the positive teaching points in your story.

- Use "analogue markings" to highlight specific learnings for the Unconscious Mind. This mean that at certain parts of the story you use a certain tone of voice and perhaps also a certain gesture, or tilt your head in a certain way, or look in a certain direction, in order to mark out specifically that part of the story or those particular words. These analogue markings will not be detected by the Conscious Mind, while the Unconscious Mind will be able to pick them up.
- Never explain your metaphor! Let the metaphor be completely for the Unconscious Mind, so never explain for the Conscious Mind. You may want to use overlapping metaphors to induce trance and overwhelm the Conscious Mind.

    1. **Simplest forms of metaphors – quotes** (such as, "I went on holiday and met a woman who said …").
    2. **Isomorphic metaphors**. This is when you take a real situation with real people and apply it to a story. To create an isomorphic metaphor within an NLP context you identify the principal characters, then create a context into which you can map these characters. If you want to deepen the trance further, you also tell a story and inside the story have someone tell you a story that someone else had told him. Pace the story in such a way that the Conscious Mind of the client becomes overwhelmed, while the Unconscious Mind knows the relationship of the characters. You can also think of what the deep meaning of your metaphor is and what the key components/characters are. Then you find what you can use as symbols for these components/characters, and if you want to make sure that these symbols definitely cannot be identified by the Conscious Mind, then you find, in turn, what can be used as a symbol for the symbol, if you see what I mean.

	Map across	Map across
Character 1	Symbol A	Symbol A2
Character 2	Symbol B	Symbol B2

For example, you may want to tell a story about how you can heal anything, and the key components are a client who is very frightened because he has been told he has cancer and he is not sure whether he can heal it. Now your deep meaning may be that you want him to realize the power of his own mind and the power of love. A symbol for the client may be a man and a symbol for cancer may be a vicious dog. Another symbol for a man may be a child, while another symbol for a vicious dog may be a wolf.

Character 1: Client   Symbol A: Man   Symbol B: Child
Character 2: Cancer   Symbol A: Vicious dog Symbol B: Wolf

So you can then create a story such as the following:

A young child felt very lost and worried. She did not know how she could get home safely because there was a vicious wolf at large in the deep, wild, dark forest. She felt completely lost, frightened and sad. She knew she had to walk home, but her fear paralyzed her. However, she was very brave and determined to overcome this fear, so she started walking and it did not take long before she crossed paths with the wolf. It started snarling at her and the little girl at first did not know what to do. Then she remembered what her mother had said; all wolves can smell your fear and they are attracted by that. If you, instead, send it love, it will feel that, too. So the little girl decided to send love to the wolf from deep inside her heart, and as she did this the wolf stopped snarling and it looked at her, as if to say, "Thank you for loving me. That is all I needed." And then it vanished, without a trace. All that was left was the little girl filled with love, with a smile on her face, walking happily on her chosen path home.

3. **Naturalistic metaphors**. Ask yourself: "Where am I?" (Present state) "Where do I want to be?" (End state) "What is the process needed to get me from the present state to the end state?" Weave that into your story.

4. **Spontaneous metaphors offered by the client**. Use any metaphor given by the client to offer suggestions. For example, one woman felt that her depression was like a man in a hood sitting on her shoulders, stopping her from moving forward. I then used this metaphor to

get her to talk to the man in the hood, to see what his message and Positive Learnings were for her and then see him change and transform them into something that would help her on her journey through life. He changed into a wise old man walking ahead of her, guiding her on her path. After we had done this, her depression started to ease immediately.

5. **Living metaphors**. These are ways of delivering a compelling message directly through action. The fall of the Berlin Wall is one powerful living metaphor, as is your own life. If you want to truly change someone, then change yourself. When they see you happy and fulfilled, having been able to transform your own life, this acts as a powerful living metaphor that, indeed, it can be done.

Metaphors: nested loops

In the nested loops technique for using metaphors, you start Metaphor 1, but don't finish it, then you start Metaphor 2 and don't finish it, start Metaphor 3 and don't finish it, start Metaphor 4 and don't finish it, and once you have gone through all your metaphors in this way, you then have a break. What you have done now is set up nested loops of unfinished metaphors, which will take your client into a deep, deep level of trance.

After that, you then finish your last metaphor, then the second last one, then the one before that, and so on, all the way back to the beginning (see diagram, below). When you do this you close the loops and bring the client out of trance. You don't have to close the loops, by the way. You can just let the client be in a deep trance. This is, of course, what happens when we watch a film that has an open rather than a closed ending.

Open the loops   **Close the loops**
Metaphor 1   **Metaphor 1**
  Metaphor 2   **Metaphor 2**
    Metaphor 3   **Metaphor 3**
      Metaphor 4   **Metaphor 4**
        Metaphor 5   **Metaphor 5**
                Break

Chapter 11
Advanced Linguistics
to Affect Time

Now we are going to cover various linguistics that affect our internal representation of time. These are extremely useful when working with others, as such linguistics will help literally to break the hold the problem has on their experience of their life, as well as helping to cement their Positive Learnings in their experience of their future. This helps to fill up their convincer (the part of them that has to be convinced in order for doubt not to take over) that the problem has gone and the solutions are here to stay, as well as helping them to let go of doubt (that old companion, a little rascal). We all have doubt. It is part of the mind and the only way to let go of it is to prove to it that change is, indeed, possible. And the only way to prove this is by using time, since by seeing the effects of the change with the proof of time, doubt starts to diminish. You can help others with this by using linguistics to affect time.

Temporal submodalities to affect time – verb tense

Imagine now that you have a timeline that stretches out into the past in one direction and out into the future in another direction, and "now" is in the middle (see below).

Past ————————————— Now ————————————— Future

When you read the following sentences I want you to notice what happens inside your mind. Be aware of where on your internal timeline you place each sentence:
1. You are changing now.
2. You have changed.

3. You will change.
4. You have had many changes.
5. You will have made many changes.
6. You had made many changes.
7. Having made many changes you decided to change.

Examples of using linguistic submodalities to shift time

Think of a time when you hadn't learnt something yet and as you look back on that time now, you realize how you eventually did learn what you needed to. Remember how you used to feel when you were little and wanted to learn how to ride a bike, and as you look back on that time now, you realize how easy it was for you to learn how to do it, and now your body does it automatically. This is how easy it is to learn new things, with time; it will all be second nature and then when you look back on now you realize how much you have learnt already, haven't you?

Another example: You may already have made all the changes you need to make now, and before you allow them to integrate fully here, in this instant, what are the other Positive Learnings and insights, some other positive resources, you can add to this change now, to make it even deeper, even more transformative? And you can allow these learnings, insights and resources to come up within your Unconscious Mind in an instant, or maybe even quicker than that, and notice how much you are changing on every level now, and how it fills your whole being with resources, and know deep within you how this will happen all by itself, just as it is happening right now, isn't it?

Aligning intention

The premise with this is that when we create positive experiences and results in our lives it will be because the underlying intention is positive and based in love. When we create negative experiences in our lives it is because the underlying intention is negative, fearful and less resourceful.
- So think of something that is a problem in your life.
- I want you now to float back into the past to the first event, when you first had that thought that created this problem in your life.

- And go now to just before that.
- Now, as you are here, just before this event, just notice what your original intention was for choosing to perceive the event in this way – the original intent behind that first thought. Is the intent positive or negative?
- Now I want you to notice what would happen if you instead chose a truly Positive Intention, an intention based in love? How would you choose to think then? How would that change how you perceive this event? Notice what would happen in your life if you were to choose to act on this Positive Intention based in love instead – and do that all the way back from that first event to now.
- Think of that old problem and notice how you feel now.
- Now look forward to the future and notice how much better you feel now, when you allow your intention to be coming from a place of love.

Future soul sourcing

Time often heals. When it does we have moved on, learnt and changed at an inner level, and this has allowed us to redirect the focus in our lives.

Time is an illusion, albeit a very real illusion, but time is a metaphor. It does not exist at the level of real experience. The past, present and future are happening simultaneously. This is something we know about because of studies in metaphysics, and something mystics and esoteric traditions have been teaching for thousands of years. The past, present and future are treated cybernetically by the brain, and with that I mean the Unconscious Mind.

You know that time heals and you also know that there have been times in the past when you found something difficult to do, but over time you learnt to do it. And you learnt to do it when you got the learnings, insights and wisdom you needed.

Future soul sourcing process

(This is available to be downloaded at www.nordiclightinstitute.com)

What I want you to do now is to close your eyes and imagine you are floating above the present moment and float way, way up into the sky, up to a beautiful, sacred mountain top, so you can clearly see your own life down there: your past and your future. As you are sitting up here on this beautiful mountain top, I want you to invite your most evolved Higher Self, to be up here with you. Together, look down on your life down there and notice a problem that you are currently encountering and which you would now like to solve and heal.

Then ask your Higher Self what the Positive Learnings are for you, so that you can heal this now? What other Positive Learnings are there?

What is it your Higher Self wants you to know and learn so you can heal this now? What is it your Higher Self wants you to pay attention to so you can heal this now? What does your Higher Self want you to focus on so you can do that?

What I want you to do now is to take your Higher Self's hand and let your Higher Self float up with you from this sacred mountain and instead float all the way out into the future, to a time when you have learnt all the future Positive Learnings, insights and wisdom you need for you to heal this fully now. So float out into the future to the point where you have learnt all these learnings, insight and wisdom. Just keep moving toward the future until you have learnt what you need to learn, and as you are learning this, your Unconscious Mind is learning all of this, too, because it remembers everything.

Now when you are enriched with your new learnings, insights and wisdom, notice how much you have changed. How are you feeling now?

As you are feeling _____ [stated Positive Emotion], turn around and look at the past and bring all your resources, insights, learnings and wisdom all the way back to now, only as quickly as your Unconscious Mind realigns your past in light of your new choices, learnings and wisdom, focusing on what is really important in your life, now and in the future.

As you look toward the future now, what is important to you now?

Now go out into the future and notice how you are being, doing and having – thanks to your learnings, insights and wisdom.

Come back to now and thank your Higher Self for doing this work with you.

Chapter 12
Advanced Linguistic Reframes

Inductive and deductive language patterns

It is extremely important to know about these language patterns, for reasons that will become clear.

A deductive statement is: "Since I never liked learning foreign languages at school, I will never be able to learn a foreign language."

Here you take one statement and use it to limit your options by applying it in a limiting way to other examples, and in this way you are limiting your experience.

An inductive statement is: "If I can learn to do this, I can learn to do anything."

This pattern will help to blow out the boundary (break through the boundary of the problem), because you are breaking the statement outward (the statement in itself is "expanding").

So here you take one statement and you use it to expand your options, and in this way you are expanding your experience.

Non-mirror image reverse inductive language pattern

Boundary condition in the nervous system

I remember being on my Master Practitioner's course and how using this language pattern effectively blew the boundary pattern (which expands, so has to "blow out" the boundary with its expansion) of one of my problems. It was incredible and since then I have used it often.

The way this is used is as follows. You have a Problem Boundary, such as a Problem Strategy (see pages 112–16) or a Prime Concern (see pages 121–2). To blow out the boundary you use an inductive language pattern, and you also blow it out by taking the non-mirror image reverse of the problem (which will obviously lie outside the boundary, as it is the opposite to the problem). This will seem easier once I have gone through a few examples, so just bear with me on this one.

You can run the language pattern as a question expressed as, **"It is not just about (the opposite of the problem) though, isn't it?"** ("Isn't it" may be grammatically incorrect, but it is correct in this NLP context, and it helps to induce trance mode.) For example, say someone is feeling unable to commit in a relationship, you say,

"It is not just about commitment in a relationship, though, isn't it?"

Now this sentence will not make sense to anyone who has not got the problem, but when you start to hit the boundary of someone's problem it will make sense to them, so that they start to say things like, "Yes, that's right", or "Yes", or "No, I know", or a similar response and they will start to get a really trance-like look, and then you'll know you are on the right track. So you just keep repeating the same question over and over again, as many as five to nine times, until they, in a way, cannot hear you, and what you are saying to them completely makes sense, at which point you start to calibrate a physiological shift.

Another way of generating an inductive language pattern is when you get a problem expressed as a Cause and Effect. You then chunk up (see page 109) on the effect, until you find the non-mirror image reverse (the opposite of the problem), and then you use this non-mirror image reverse in a language pattern expressed as, **"Anything less than the total opposite of (the problem) isn't (the non mirror-image reverse) though, isn't it?"** For example, someone feels they are unacceptable because they feel they are unlovable. When you chunk up on the word "unlovable", by asking what is the highest intention, the highest purpose, you may end up getting to love (which is the non-mirror image reverse of unlovable); you can then use it in a question such as:

"So anything less than total acceptance isn't love, though, isn't it?

"So anything less than total love isn't acceptance, though, isn't it?"

There is no way for you to know which sentence will work better for your particular client until you have said it and have calibrated the response in him or her.

You can also use this with a Limiting Decision. Say someone has a Limiting Decision that they can't follow their dreams, then when you chunk up on that you may get happiness, so you can then say, "So anything less than totally following your dreams isn't happiness, though, isn't it?"

You can also swap the words around and say, "So anything less than total happiness isn't following your dreams, though, isn't it?"

Or if someone has a problem letting go of sadness and you chunk up on "sadness", you might get happiness (which is the non-mirror image reverse, that is, the opposite), so you can say, "So anything less than totally letting go of this sadness isn't happiness, though, isn't it?"

It is a bit like you knowing all the specific words you can use and then throwing them up in the air and just noticing how they fall when they land.

Also with these statements you keep repeating the statement over and over again until the client can't hear you, or until they just let go of their problem!

Before you say your question/statement you also say, "I want you to fully consider this – and then say your chosen statement."

Sleight of Mouth

A client I saw some time ago said she just could not forgive her father as he had hurt her too much. She suffered from severe depression, felt an immense pain in her heart and was unable to feel any happiness. So I asked her, "Would it not be easier for you to let go of this old pain and feel happy again when you have forgiven your father?"

"Oh, no," she said. "I can't do that. I don't want to give him that victory."

So I said, "What happened, happened in the past, so he is not hurting you any more is he? Instead, you are hurting yourself, because you have to live with your own thoughts and you are the one that is now holding on to the pain. For what purpose would you want to do that? Have you ever considered that not forgiving him is what causes you to still feel that old pain? Holding on to the idea that you can't forgive him will continue to hurt you forever. How much more hurting do you have to do before you can let it go? I also want you to consider that being hurt is not the real issue here. The real issue is whether you want to be happy and live your own life or be stuck in the past. Isn't it better to be happy and forgive, than hold on to old wounds? Many people feel that they can't forgive someone because they have hurt them too much, and that is because they have not yet realized how much pain this belief is causing them and how much it is costing them – in the form of losing vital Life Energy every day, Life Energy that you could instead use to create the life you want. In my experience, I have discovered that forgiveness is a gift you give yourself, not the other person, because it frees you from the past. So then the victory is yours – the victory to live your life free from the past."

My client thought about this and then, suddenly, her Unconscious Mind could see the logic in this, that, yes indeed, she was mainly hurting herself by holding on to this old pain, and that letting it go was a gift she gave to herself, not a gift she gave to her dad. Releasing her depression and old pain was, from that moment, pretty easy and she skipped out of the clinic room after her Break-Through session.

What we are going to do now is Sleight of Mouth, taken from the expression "sleight of hand", which is when a magician seems to be creating magic with his hands. In Sleight of Mouth you appear to be creating magic with the way you use words.

As you probably know by now, all our thoughts and actions are undertaken within a frame of reference (of which we may or may not be conscious). In fact, most of our thoughts and actions are driven by the Unconscious Mind. Sometimes these frames lock us into restrictive thinking that limits our choices in life. Using reframes (trying on a different frame of reference), we can assist ourselves and others to get a different perspective on a problem and other possible solutions. Reframing by itself seldom resolves the problem. Reframing offers the potential of "softening up" the problem so that its resolution is more plausible. You have already learnt about context and meaning reframes and reframe with the highest intention. Sleight of Mouth was developed by Robert Dilts through modelling the verbal patterns of people such as Karl Marx, Milton Erickson, Abraham Lincoln, Jesus and Gandhi.

As you may have already realized, Sleight of Mouth and all reframes have to be used with compassion. If you take Sleight of Mouth out of context it can come across as being very harsh, but this is not the intention. As a practitioner you have to use your language in such a way that you help your client expand their model of the world, so that they can find the inner resources they need to create a positive change in their lives.

Sleight of Mouth patterns work well for belief change. To use these patterns the client's belief must be expressed in terms of a Complex Equivalence or Cause and Effect assertion (see page 130). The statement, "I don't believe in healing," does not reveal the full belief and gives us little to work with. To ascertain the person's full belief, you could ask questions such as, "What does healing mean to you?", "What are the consequences of healing or not healing?", "What will a healing lead to?" If your client responds with a Complex Equivalence or Cause and Effect, then you have something to work with.

Sleight of Mouth patterns

a) **"I am too old to change."**
b) **"I can't forgive him, because he hurt me too much."**

1. **Intention**. What could be the Positive Intention?
   Questions you can ask yourself to help you find the suitable Sleight of Mouth response are, "Why are they saying this?", "What is the Secondary Gain?" and "What are they trying to get?"
   a) "What change is it you don't want to do, which you have to do, when you let go of the excuse?" (Secondary Gain)
   b) "Would it not be easier for you to let go of the hurt and feel happy again when you have forgiven him?"

2. **Redefine**. Use words or statements that are similar but that may imply something different.
   Question you can also ask yourself for this, before you say your Sleight of Mouth response is: "What other meaning could the Cause and Effect or Complex Equivalence statement have?"
   a) "With age comes maturity and wisdom, and with wisdom comes an abilty to change far more easily."

b) "What happened, happened in the past, so he is not hurting you any more. You are hurting yourself, because you are holding on to that old pain."

3. **Consequences**. Focus on a consequence that leads to challenging the belief.

   Question you can also ask yourself here is: "What will happen to them if they continue to think this way?"

a) "Change is inevitable, and the more you resist it, the more frustrated you will be."

b) "Holding on to that old pain will stop you from feeling happy now."

4. **Chunk down**. Look at a specific element that challenges the belief. This causes your client to have to go inside and find the specifics for why they believe that.

   Questions you can ask yourself are: "What specifically?", "What are examples of this?", "What are parts of this?"

a) "When specifically do we stop changing? Is there a particular age when that happens?"

b) "Which specific aspect of the hurt do you want to hold on to and what specifically does it give you?"

5. **Chunk up**. Generalize in order to change the relationship defined by the belief and use exaggeration.

   Questions you can ask yourself are: "For what purpose?", "What's important about this?"

a) "So do you mean people can only change while they are babies and as soon as they grow older change stops?" (Exaggeration) Or, "For what purpose do you believe people change less as they get older?"

b) "Isn't it about time you free your mind from this pain, and instead chose to be happy?"

6. **Counter example**. Find an exception that challenges the generalization defined by the belief.

   Questions you can ask yourself about this to invert the belief, and make it into a universal statement or question are: "Was there ever a time when the result (B) led to the cause (A)? Or a time when the cause (A) did not lead to the result (B)? Or perhaps a time when the opposite to the result (not B) did lead to the opposite of the cause (not A)?"

a) "Have you ever known of an older person who was able to change?"

b) "Not forgiving him is what causes you to still feel the pain."

7. **Analogy**. Use an analogy or metaphor that challenges the belief.

a) Louise Hay was in her forties when her husband left her. By 58 she had self-published her first book, which during the first year only made a $5 profit. But by the time she was 85, her book *You Can Heal Your Life* had sold over 45 million copies! She still sees life as a great adventure. When she turned 80 she said to herself: "Louise, this is going to be the best decade of your life!" And, according to her, it is.

b) When I forgave my dad, I could feel how a huge weight lifted from my whole being. I was suddenly filled with light, happiness and a sense of expansion. It was the greatest gift I could ever have given to myself, because I had freed myself to create a happy life.

8. **Apply to Self**. Use key aspects of the belief to challenge it. When you ask yourself a question about it you don't think about it, but just apply it back on to itself.

a) "What age were you when you stopped changing?"

b) "Holding on to that belief will continue to hurt you forever. How much more hurting do you have to do before you can let it go?"

9. **Another outcome**. Propose a different outcome that challenges the relevance of the belief.

a) "The question here has nothing to do with change, and instead more to do with whether you are old enough to allow wisdom to be your agent of change."

b) "Being hurt is not the real issue here. The real issue is whether you want to be happy and live your own life, or be stuck in the past."

10. **Hierarchy of criteria**. Reassess the belief based on a more important criterion.

a) "How would it be if you were to focus on how much you have grown and changed already instead of how old you are?"

b) "Isn't it better to be happy and forgive, than to hold on to old wounds?"

11. Change frame size. Re-evaluate the belief in the context of a longer (or shorter) time frame, a larger number of people (or from an individual point of view) or a bigger (or smaller) perspective.

Aspects for this that you can consider are: something larger or smaller they have not noticed; different frame, same behaviour; chunk up on universal quantifier (see page 130).

a) "If no one was able to change with age, society would never evolve."

b) "If you were to hold on to all past hurt you would never be able to move forward and be happy and mature in wisdom."

12. Meta Frame. Challenge the basis for the belief. For example, formulate a belief as to the origin of the belief.

The question for this that you ask yourself can be: "How is it possible they can believe that?"

a) "That's because you haven't yet noticed the link between growing in maturity and wisdom and age."

b) "Many people feel that they can't forgive someone because they have hurt them too much, and that's because they have not yet realized how much pain this belief is causing them."

13. Model of the World. Look at the belief from a different perspective (model of the world).

a) "In many other cultures you gain respect and status the older you are, because it is known that with age comes wisdom, and with wisdom comes the ability to change."

b) "In my experience, I have discovered that when people forgive, they free themselves from the bondage of the past, so forgiveness is a gift you give yourself, not a gift you give to the other person."

14. Reality strategy. Reassess the belief based on the fact that beliefs are based on specific perceptions.

Questions you can ask yourself are: "How do they represent that belief and how do they know if it is not true?"

a) "Can you be absolutely sure that belief is true?"

b) "How would you know what happens to your old hurt when you forgive, if you don't try it?"

If you now look at any of your Limiting Beliefs, Prime Concerns or similar, and state them as a Cause and Effect sentence (tip: use the word "because"), or as a Complex Equivalence (tip: use the words "am", "is", "means"), then you will be able to come up with your own Sleight of Mouth patterns to reframe your own Unconscious Mind!

Summary of the linguistic patterns

It is surprising how you can use language to facilitate healing and how you can use it to shift someone's Internal Representation, so you can assist them in creating positive Internal Representations, which will serve them, helping them achieve the results they want. And the best part about linguistics is that you can use it at any time, with anyone – with your friends, your family, your boss, your colleagues, your in-laws – anyone. So you can be like an Angel Coach in disguise, helping your clients to find more resources within themselves, without them knowing that this is what you are doing.

So learn your linguistic skills as well as you can and you will then be able to facilitate deep healing in others and yourself. Trust your Unconscious Mind. It is so much wiser than you could ever imagine. Just think about what is required of your Unconscious Mind to make your heart beat, allow your lungs to breathe. Imagine what is required of it to learn how to speak, how to walk and skip and how to get on with others. Wonderful skills, so trust it now too, that if it can do that, then it can also learn how to use all these fantastic language patterns, so that one day, perhaps today or tomorrow, or some other time in the future, or perhaps even quicker than that, you will look back on today and realize that your Unconscious Mind has known these patterns all along, that in fact it cannot not know them, because they are now deeply embedded within your Unconscious Mind.

If you want to learn more linguistics, I recommend David Shepherd's *Conversational Change* from www.performancepartnership.com

PART 4

Developing Wisdom and Increasing Your Spiritual Energy

Chapter 13
Developing Wisdom

Developing inner balance and wisdom is a vital skill to master, and for you to be able to do this you have to be willing to work on yourself so you are able to heal yourself and your life.

One of the most fundamental practices for developing a balanced mind is meditation, as this helps you to still your own frantic thoughts. If you just meditate 10 minutes a day you will notice positive results and if you can meditate 20 minutes per day, you will receive even greater rewards. Meditation allows you to connect with a wise, still aspect of yourself and once you have learnt to connect with it, you can then receive answers and solutions to your own problems and dilemmas in life far more easily. Meditation becomes your inner compass and guiding light.

How can meditation help you achieve balance?

Dr Daniel Siegel writes in his book *The Mindful Brain* how research has found, through the study of MRI scans, that the prefrontal cortex area of the brain (behind our forehead) becomes more developed in people who meditate every day. This area of the brain is responsible for empathy, compassion, the ability to tune in to others and perception. Our pre-frontal area is not fully developed until we are 25 years of age.

We are all born with our primitive area of the brain functioning well. This area deals with our fear, anger, survival and our insistence in winning an argument. As we move through childhood and adulthood we learn more and more, and we start to react more with our prefrontal area instead of our more primitive brain. Meditation helps us to do this even more effectively. An interesting note is that in yoga philosophy, which dates back thousands of years, the forehead area (our third eye) is seen as the seat of our heightened consciousness, and the back of our head (where the primitive brain is roughly situated), the seat of our ego. Science is slowly catching up with ancient esoteric teachings!

Neurological motorway

The more you use certain pathways in the brain, the more neurological connections are formed. It is as though you create a motorway out of a particular thought pathway. This means that if you often think fearful thoughts, your fearful brain pathways become wider and more developed; it's rather like creating a Motorway of Fear. Similarly, if you often think loving thoughts, these loving pathways become wider and more developed, creating a Motorway of Love, helping you to connect with your loving thoughts more easily and quickly.

David Hamilton, PhD, writes in his book *Why Kindness is Good for You* about how scientists have found that thinking the same kinds of thoughts over and over again causes structural changes in the brain.

Meditation helps you to develop the prefrontal cortex area of your brain, enabling you to feel more empathy, be more balanced and more perceptive of others. It also helps you to control your thoughts and let go of fear and instead focus on love and happiness. This helps you to form new, loving and happy neurological pathways in your brain, making it easier for you to be loving and happy in your daily life.

Some simple meditation techniques

Peripheral vision and Ha Breathing

Focus on a spot straight ahead of you. As you focus on it, also expand your awareness to the periphery and then expand it even further behind you, while still focusing on the spot ahead. You are now in peripheral vision, which stills your nervous system (increases the parasympathetic system and shuts down your sympathetic system).

Breathe in through your nose and out through your mouth, making the sound "Haaaa" as you breathe out. Carry on at your own pace while focusing on the spot and with your awareness of the periphery and behind you. After a while you may want to close your eyes while still performing the Ha Breathing.

Meditation for letting go and finding the stillness within

Sit or lie down comfortably. Feel whether there is any tension in your body. Increase the tension as you breathe in and as you breathe out let the tension go. Keep doing this with any area of your body where you experience tension. Then do the same with your mind. Feel whether there is any tension in your mind, increase it as you breathe in and as you breathe out let the tension go. Now see whether there is anything or anyone you are feeling tense about. Increase the tension as you breathe in, and as you breathe out imagine cutting the cords (you can do this with an imaginary sword or scissors) and let the tension go. Keep doing this with anything you feel tense about. Then imagine a healing fire is circling all around you, burning away any old tension, cleansing you, leaving you totally free, relaxed and still. Now sink deep into the stillness within you. Flow deeper and deeper, sinking more and more into the stillness. Let it surround you, filling every cell of your being. Now flow inside your heart and give thanks and gratitude for all that is positive and helpful in your life.

Our inner energy

It is really important to have strong inner energy, since you use it to create your life. Also, if you have less energy than others, you may start "feeding" off other people's energy instead of using your own inner energy to help yourself. The following is an overview of how we lose energy and how we can increase our inner energy.

- **Engaging in negative thoughts and emotions** is the most effective way of decreasing your body's energy levels. Sadness, guilt and depression, by their very nature, tend to decrease your energy levels; and anger, fear and anxiety increase your sympathetic nervous system response, which leads first to an increased sense of energy, only later to crash and leave you feeling depleted. Negative emotions will, in the end, always lead to a decrease of your available inner energy.
- **Thinking about "negative" events that happened in the past** eats up a lot of available energy. The further back the event is, the more energy you have to invest in it, in order for it to be able to remain "alive" in your mind. If something happened yesterday, it is less of

an effort to make that memory "alive" in your mind than if the event happened in your childhood. Worrying about the future also eats up energy, as does worrying about money. Escaping into a fantasy world by dreaming too much about the future (without following up with appropriate action to make it real), or watching too much TV, can also eat away at the energy you have in the present moment.

- **Repressed emotional pain now manifesting as physical pain** is another common finding. When something happens to you that you, at the time, are not able to deal with, your Unconscious Mind represses the content and emotions of this situation. Because your Unconscious Mind also runs your body and it takes up a lot of energy to keep memories repressed, less energy will then be available for use by the body. This is logical. Now, if the Unconscious Mind has to keep these memories repressed for a long time, they will often start to be mirrored within your body as pain and discomfort. Therefore, any chronic pain you are having may have an emotional component to it, and often this is the case in acute pain as well.

- **Giving your power away**, either by relying too much on others (what they think, what they want you to do, or letting them help you out too much), or by focusing more on taking responsibility for other people's lives, instead of dealing with, and taking responsibility for, your own life.

- **Any obsession** you have, whether about food, exercise, money, work, a hobby or even a person, will lead to decreased health. Why? Because obsession is a clear indicator that your thoughts are not in balance, and therefore it will bring with it many negative thoughts and emotions. This is why diets don't work. The more you deny yourself certain foods, the more you become obsessed with them. This is because you are focusing on everything that you can't have, and so the mind constantly keeps thinking about it. As long as you are forcing yourself consciously to control your urges *not* to eat certain foods, you will succeed in your chosen diet. As soon as you stop, guess what happens? You immediately want to eat the things you formerly denied yourself. Then you beat yourself up about it, which leads to even more negative thoughts and emotions! Also,

175

when you are dieting your body realizes that it is being starved and therefore it holds on to fat and only loses water, because it knows it may take a while for it to receive proper energy again and fat is a great source of energy. During a diet your body also slows down your metabolism, making it even harder for you to lose weight. The moment you stop your diet, you put the weight back on, but this time with even more fat, because your body remembers that you recently starved it. It stores extra fat, just in case. It wants to protect you and it does not want you to starve yourself to death.

- It's easy to be obsessive about exercise and this is clearly visible in some exercise fanatics. They may be physically strong, but they worry and constantly think about exercise, whether they look good, whether they are strong enough, whether they are good enough the way they are. An obsession with exercise may also be a sign that there are unhealed emotions within the Unconscious Mind that the person does not want to pay attention to, and in order not to have to deal with it, the person becomes fanatical about exercise. Other people use different obsessive strategies, such as working all the time or overindulging in smoking, alcohol and drugs.

- The same applies to most other forms of health fanaticism. When you obsess about a health problem, you will automatically worry about it, whether you have it or not. So you can't win. Give up fanatical behaviour and instead allow yourself to be in balance.

- You can also be obsessed by certain thought patterns or behaviours, believing that somehow they will give you peace and calm.

- **Worrying about what other people might think of you** is another way in which you can lose energy. Just remember, what other people think of you is none of your business!

The following Life-Energy Test has been inspired by the work of Caroline Myss on Energy Medicine.

Life-Energy Test

Imagine waking up each morning to a magical pot of 100 golden coins for you to use as Life Energy during the day. These are yours to use as you wish; yours to use as energy to manifest the life you want. Let us now see how much of this energy is stolen and used up by the common energy thieves. For every question below, just go with the first figure that pops into your head and write it down immediately.

1. How much Life Energy do you use up in negative thinking every day, such as negative thoughts about yourself, other people or events from your past? From 0 to 100 coins? Your answer: _____

2. How much Life Energy do you use up in worrying about the future? From 0 to 100 coins? Your answer: _____

3. How much Life Energy do you use up in worrying about money? From 0 to 100 coins? Your answer: _____

4. How much Life Energy do you use up in dreaming about the future (without taking action to fulfil your dreams) or in watching too much TV? From 0 to 100 coins? Your answer: _____

5. How much energy do you use up by repressing emotional pain? From 0 to 100 coins? Your answer: _____

6. How much Life Energy do you lose by giving your power away? From 0 to 100 coins? Your answer: _____

7. How much Life Energy is used up by any obsession you have? From 0 to 100 coins? Your answer: _____

8. How much Life Energy do you use up by worrying about what other people might think? From 0 to 100 coins? Your answer: _____

- Life Energy left over if your start-up sum is 100 golden coins: _____ (this could be + or –)

How we can incur an energy debt

For some people total "spending" may be higher than the daily magical pot of golden coins. This means that every day, the available energy you have to spend is not enough to fund your habits of wasting energy by engaging in negative thinking, holding on to past negative events, worrying about the future, worrying about money, escaping into fantasy land by losing yourself in dreams about the future or watching too much TV, repressing emotional pain held in the body, giving your power away, investing energy in various obsessions or worrying about what others might think of you. This means that you start to incur an "energy debt", which you then have to start paying back. Since you may not have any money to pay it back with, you incur even more debt. You then start to look for ways of borrowing Life Energy, and the first place the Unconscious Mind borrows from is the body. Then you wonder why you are so tired and why you do not have the energy to change your life. The Unconscious Mind can also borrow energy from other people, or by choosing to get worked up with stress or drink gallons of coffee to get the adrenaline flowing and in this way give you momentary energy. All of this will lead to even more exhaustion.

As you start to address this energy imbalance, as you start to heal, you may still have an energy debt to pay back, so some of your golden coins will have to be used to pay off your debt. This can take time. If you then start to worry or get frustrated about why it seems to take so long, then you again start to eat into your available gold coins of Life Energy to spend every day. However, if you continue to work on yourself, disciplining your mind and learning to stop wasting your energy in negativity, or by focusing too much on your past or your future, thereby missing the present moment, then after a while your debt will have been paid back and you will be able to use all your available gold coins as Life Energy to fund all the dreams that you want to manifest into reality. This is when things start to happen really quickly: you are able to have an idea, a divine guidance, make the choice to follow it and take action to follow it, and very quickly it manifests in your physical reality.

Is it possible to wipe out an energy debt?

Yes. When you completely forgive everyone, including yourself, when you let go of your past, when you accept everything that has happened and everything that is happening, when you have faith and trust in the Divine and stop trying to be in control, when you live your life fully as you, being authentic with who you are, allowing your spiritual energy to be expressed fully through you, as you, then all your energy debt is instantaneously wiped out. For example, an NLP Transformational Break-Through Healing Session can help you to wipe this debt clean, as can many other forms of therapies, such as Shamanic Soul Journeying.

Once the debt has been wiped out, however, you then have to continue mastering your own energy by not allowing it to be invested in negativity, which could then start to create a new debt. From time to time, take the Life-Energy Test in order to establish how much of your Life Energy you have available to use each day.

Like attracts like

Any Life Energy you have, you will invest. When you invest in negative actions, thoughts and behaviours, negative energy flows out from you into the world and it then later comes back as a negative energy return, increasing your Life-Energy debt. Since like energy attracts like energy you will here draw to you more negative experiences. This is negative karma.

When you, instead, take actions fuelled with positive thoughts and emotions and with a positive attitude, this positive energy will flow out from you into the world, and it will also come back to you as a positive energy return. Since like energy attracts like energy you will here draw to you more positive experiences. When you use your Life Energy wisely and invest it in that which will be for the highest good of everyone, it will return to you multiplied. This is how you create positive karma.

Additional tips for increasing your energy

It is important to look after your physical energy. When our bodies are healthy it is easier for us to feel happy and optimistic, so make sure you:

- Get enough sleep.
- Eat a diet that is in tune with your intuition (preferably organic and as natural as possible).
- Allow your body to exercise regularly (for example, through Zumba, Pilates, yoga, dancing or walking).
- Make sure your body gets the holistic treatment it needs (for example, through osteopathy, chiropractic, naturopathy, herbs, craniosacral therapy, acupuncture, Ayurvedic medicine or massage).

Chapter 14
Preparing for the Transformational Break-Through Healing Session

Before we start the deeply healing Transformational Break-Through Session I want to outline a few important pointers that are useful to bear in mind throughout the process.

The Wounded Self and the Wise Inner Self

Remember the difference between the Wounded Self and the Wise Inner Self, which both reside in the Unconscious Mind (see page 28)? When you are working with yourself both aspects can be talking to you, and it is important to be able to distinguish which is which.

First, let me explain a bit more about these two. The Wounded Self is linked to the fearful inner ego – our inner darkness – and the Wise Inner Self is linked to our higher, Divine Self, our higher, conscious awareness, our inner light. Remember that these are just metaphors used to explain an energy.

Our negative inner programming will be from the Wounded Self and what heals negative inner programming is the wisdom communicated to us from the Wise Inner Self. Every time we take steps to heal this negative inner programming, we dive deep within our inner darkness, bringing the light from our Wise Inner Selves with us, like a divine torch, and we transform the old darkness into light. This causes us to feel lighter, to be lighter and to shine even more brightly.

Let's say that you take yourself through a Transformational Break-Through Healing Session and you release a Problem Strategy, you will float above the event and can then ask for the Positive Learnings. You then state these Positive Learnings in the following form: "They did not mean to hurt me", "I do not have to care that they dislike me", "I am not alone", "I can just ignore them", "I can walk away".

When you look at these learnings you can see that they are not of a very high Logical Level (see pages 107–11), in that they are not strong enough to create a healing, and they are still looking at the event through wounded eyes, so it is the Wounded Self that is speaking. When that happens I just keep asking, "So what are the other Positive Learnings here for you?"

Eventually you will start to state Positive Learnings that are of a higher Logical Level, that is of a sufficiently high quality to be able to create a healing shift in the client. Examples of such Positive Learnings are, "Love is all around us", "They do love me", "I can follow my dreams", "The power to change my life is within me".

Notice that these Positive Learnings are powerful. They come from the Wise Inner Self, which is able to receive clear communication from your Higher Consciousness, that is your Higher Self. I always write these Positive Learnings down. I never write down the statements from the Wounded Self, only from the Wise Inner Self.

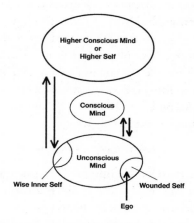

The metaphor of the ego is our inner darkness, which communicates with the Wounded Self. The metaphor of our Higher Conscious Mind, our Higher Self, communicates with our Wise Inner Self.

In my model of the world, I feel that in a Healing Break-Through session, all we do is enable ourselves to connect more fully with our divine inner light, power and resources, and by doing this we are able to let go of the grip the inner ego has on us. The ego talks to us through the Wounded Inner Self. So what is the ego then?

The fearful ego is an illusion

The darkness, the fearful ego, is an illusion. It is not real. It may seem real at times, because we make it real when we focus our thoughts on it. We give it power by feeding it with our fear, focus and thinking. It is, however, not real. How do I know this? Simple. If it were real, then it would be what remains as you bring in the light of your Loving Soul – the light of your divine essence. And it does not stay. Instead every time, as you bring in the light, the darkness disappears. Every time, as you bring in love and wisdom, the wound within you heals. Every time.

Now remember that the ego is not real – it is an illusion. However, in our world of illusion it seems real. The ego is just the energy that separates us from the Divine and tempts us to remain locked in dense matter, by tempting us into desire, attachments, judgments and fear – all of which separate us further from the Divine, separating us from love.

I believe that we are now at a threshold where the consciousness of humanity has the chance of evolving so much that we are able to live our lives free from the ego and in this way are able to express our divinity through our lives here on Earth. This, I believe, will create the metaphor of Heaven on Earth. To do this we all have to undertake our journey of awakening to our own divinity.

How the ego is insane

I agree with Eckhart Tolle's description of how the ego is insane (read *A New Earth*). If you look at the world you can see how the ego has created a collective madness in the way we treat each other and the planet. The fearful ego will always lead you to more pain and destruction. So what makes the ego insane? It is because it is based on fear, negativity, a belief that it is separate from everyone else, a belief that it is small and insignificant, and in order to make itself feel better it will try to be superior to others, it will try to take everything it can take and it will view everything and everyone with fear, greed and mistrust.

The ego also fears that it will one day die, when your body dies and hence it fears death more than anything. It knows it is not eternal and it also knows the truth about you, which is that you are a being of light and love. It tries to trick you into believing you actually are the ego, that you are identified with your physical form and it does so by seducing you into believing that you are your name, your profession, your body, your bank account, your material possessions and so on. The more you identify with your outer life, the more trapped by the ego you are, and the more fear you will create within you, because all these outer manifestations will one day leave you. That is a fact and you are aware of this. You cannot take your money, your house, your possessions or your looks with you when you die. What you do take with you is your love, your learnings, your wisdom and your growth as a soul. Also the more you identify with your ego, by trying to find happiness outside yourself by earning more money, having a bigger house, looking stunning, being respected by others, or living your life through your work, partner or children, the more disconnected you will feel inside, because your ego disconnects you from your true nature, your divine, spiritual essence.

I feel the main reason people come to me for coaching is because they have disconnected from their true authentic selves, and all I do is coach them to let go of the grip their inner negativity, their inner ego, has on them and instead connect them more fully with their spiritual nature. I never say this to them – and if they do not believe in a spiritual dimension I use a different language with them, instead using the metaphor of thinking positively versus thinking negatively. It does not matter whether they believe in a spiritual nature or not – their souls do not get offended. Our souls always try to help us no matter what, and as soon as we invite our divine energy into our lives by focusing more on love and letting go of fear, divine magic will start to happen.

What does the ego do when you start to heal and change?

As you start to heal and change, as you start to bring in more and more light within your old darkness, the more your fearful ego loses its grip on you and the freer and lighter you feel. However, when you travel on this journey, when you bring in more light, your fearful ego will resist it at all costs. It will try every trick of the trade to convince you that it would be better for you to stay the way you were, because that, at least, you are familiar with. As the old saying goes, "Better the devil you know than the devil you don't." When that happens, and it will, know that you always have a choice! You can choose to listen to your fearful, insane ego, which will talk to you with fear, negativity, doubt, anxiety, judgment and worry, separating you from your inner light, separating you from the people you love and who love you, or you can choose to listen to the voice of your spiritual essence, which will connect you with your inner light and love and connect you with the people you love and who love you.

So your fearful ego knows it is not eternal. Your soul, on the other hand, which is the loving divine essence within you, knows it is eternal. It knows it is connected with everyone else and it also knows that the ego is completely mad and only an illusion, because the ego is not who you are. It is never your real nature – it is just the nightmare you find yourself believing in, until the moment you wake up and discover the real truth about yourself. That is why spiritual development is often called an *awakening*. In order to help you awaken, in every wound within you, in every place within your mind full of darkness, in every corner within you, which is in the hold of your fearful ego, divine spiritual wisdom has placed the greatest gift of healing. It is as though within each and every dark aspect of your mind there lies a precious diamond just waiting for the light to reach it, so that it can shine and radiate with its beauty, thereby enabling the darkness to disappear.

Remember the words from the wise Paramahansa Yogananda, "The only difference between a piece of coal and a diamond is the pressure that has been exerted on it."

Your Divine Soul uses the pressure that is being exerted on you when the ego is trying to lock you into darkness, negativity and fear. Every time you choose to listen to the loving voice from your Divine Soul instead of listening to the fearful voice from the ego, you allow this extra pressure to be exerted to polish and bring out your inner divine diamond, enabling your Divine Soul's light to shine through you and out into the world. This then becomes a gift you give to yourself and to everyone else.

So be courageous, be daring, be honest with yourself. Be willing to go into every dark corner of your mind, enabling you to find these beautiful diamonds, and by doing this you empower yourself to take action so that you are able to let your past go – starting now.

It is when you change your thoughts about the past that it stops hurting you, and it is when you change your thinking that your life changes too.

This is what you are doing during a Transformational Break-Through Healing Session. I have found it helpful to remember that everything we are releasing during the session is just an illusion and what you are really connecting with is the truth about you – and it is this truth that heals you.

Creating a sacred space for healing

You can create a sacred physical space just by finding a room where you will be undisturbed and then imagine this room is a sacred chamber, like a sacred, healing, nurturing sanctuary. Then you seal this space from any outside disturbance (put your phone on silent) and you can do this by imagining a bubble around this room – a bubble of light and healing.

PART 5

Transformational
Break-Through Healing

This part of the book takes you through a personal Transformational Break-Through Healing Session. If you wish to work with others, please read the whole of this part, as well as Part 6, where we cover more in-depth material on how to do this with someone else. If you are working with yourself, be sure to write down your answers.

Chapter 15
The Transformational Break-Through Healing Session

Think of a problem you have in your life – the biggest problem, which if healed, would transform your life. (Note that in NLP we "do" a problem, rather than "have" it, implying that we can also "do" something different.) Then answer these questions:

1. What is the problem? Can you remember a time when you did this problem? (Now find the Problem Strategy, so see the section on eliciting problem strategies, pages 112–16).
2. If I had a magic wand and waved it in the air and your problem completely disappeared, immediately, forever, how would you know that it had gone? What would you feel, see, hear, think, notice? (Elicits Solution Strategy.)
3. When do you do your problem?
4. How do you know it is time to do it?
5. When don't you do it?
6. How long have you had this problem?
7. What have you done about it so far?
8. Was there ever a time when you did not experience your problem?
9. Describe what happened the very first time you experienced this problem.
10. Is there a relationship between that first event and the problem as it is now?
11. What has happened since that first event?
12. When you think of your problem, what emotions do you feel and where in your body do you feel them? You release this later with

a Somato-Emotional Drop Down Through (outlined in the next chapter, see pages 199–207).

13. Is there a relationship between your childhood and your problem?

14. Is there a relationship between your problem and your relationship with your mother, father, siblings and any other key figure during your childhood (approach them all separately)?

15. If you were to imagine looking at yourself having this problem … What is it that you believe about yourself that is causing you to have this problem in your life? What is it that you believe that you are that is causing this problem? What do you believe about yourself or about life? (This will give you many of your Limiting Beliefs. Then look to see which three Limiting Beliefs are the main ones for you, which if you released them, your problem would disappear.)

16. Ask your Unconscious Mind what is the purpose of having this problem in your life and when did you decide to create it?

17. If there was anything your Unconscious Mind wanted you to pay attention to, such that if you were to pay attention to it your problem would completely disappear, what would it be?

18. Is there anything your Unconscious Mind wants you to know and learn, the knowing and learning about which would cause your problem to disappear?

19. What are you pretending not to know by having your problem in your life?

20. Look at what the possible outcome would be when you change this negative situation into a positive one and compare that with what would happen if you allowed the problem to stay the same. Think ahead to one year from now and notice the difference. Five years from now. Ten years from now. Do you want the problem to change? (You have to say "Yes" here!)

To find out the Secondary Gain, the "rewards", you receive from having your problem

It is important to find your Secondary Gain, so that you are aware of how attached you are to having the problem, so make sure your Positive

Learnings and Insights (which you will find later on in the intervention) are strong enough to release the Secondary Gain:

- What is this problem preventing you from doing, which if this problem disappears, you will have to do?
- What is it you are not doing because this problem is in your life?
- What is it that you are doing, which you enjoy doing that you won't be able to do when your problem disappears?
- What is it that you are not doing, that you don't want to do, that you will have to do when your problem disappears?
- Ask your Unconscious Mind if it is totally willing to assist and support you in having an undeniable experience of having this problem disappearing here when you are going through this process. (You have to say, "Yes".)
- Elicit values (see pages 119–21) for the main area you are working with. Put them in order.

The different areas for values elicitation (just choose one):

- Family
- Relationships (specify which relationship – partner, children, friends, etc)
- Work/being of service
- Health and well-being
- Personal development
- Spiritual development

Intervention

Once you have gone through the questions, transfer everything you have found onto an Intervention Document, following the guidelines below.

Higher-Self Healing (a version of this process can be downloaded from www.nordiclightinstitute.com, and you will also find it outlined on pages 194–9) to release:

1. Problem Strategy
2. Negative Emotions
   Write down all the Negative Emotions you have found.

As you release the Problem Strategies you have probably released some of these Negative Emotions, too, so if you think that has happened, then before releasing a Negative Emotion you think might have gone, ask yourself, "Is this _____ [specific Negative Emotion] still there for me, or has it now gone?"

3. Limiting Beliefs

First write down your top three Limiting Beliefs and always release the top one.

Write down ALL the Limiting Beliefs you have found during the questioning session. Remember you cannot release a Limiting Belief which has a "not" in it, as the Unconscious Mind cannot compute a negative (see page 108).

Some Limiting Beliefs may have been released by you having done the work on Problem Strategies and Negative Emotions, so here too you ask whether this specific Limiting Belief is still there or if it is now gone.

Also, if you found some major Prime Concerns (see pages 121–2) you can release these too with Higher-Self Healing.

Healing with the Highest Intention Reframe (download a version of this process from www.nordiclightinstitute.com; see also pages 95–8).
Always do this on the main problem.

Parts Integration, if needed (see pages 101–6)
Always write down all the Parts Conflicts you have identified. By the time you do the Parts Integration exercise many previous Parts Conflicts will have healed by you having done the previous work. So here, before you release a Parts Conflict ask yourself, "So how is that a problem now? How is that a conflict?"

If you say that it is not a problem any more and you calibrate that this is correct, then you know you do not need to do a Parts Integration. If you say it is still there, and/or you calibrate it is still there, then you release it.

Somato-Emotional Drop Down Through on body part associated with problem (see pages 199–207).

Forgiveness Exercise (and Perceptual Positions if needed; see pages 59–63 and 207–11).

Write down the names of all the people you need to do this with, including your parents, siblings and family, as well as other key figures

Goal-setting (see pages 211–16)
Setting goals is important to help give the Unconscious Mind a direction. Make sure the goals are stated in the positive. This will help to cement the learnings the Unconscious Mind and Wise Higher Self has given during the session.

Re-checking values (see pages 216–18)
All values have to be 100 per cent positive at the end of the session. So re-check your values here. If a value is not 100 per cent positive, then ask yourself, "As you are now, within yourself in your thoughts, having done all this work, is there anything in your thoughts that could stop you from having 100 per cent positive energy in moving toward creating this in your future now?"

When I ask clients this they realize that as they are now in their thoughts, there is nothing that can stop them from moving forward toward creating this positive value in their lives. So I then ask, "Great, so how much is that now a positive value for you?"

Final Meditation including meeting the Future You and the Solution Strategy (see pages 250–53) This will help you to make sure you are running your Solution Strategy at the end of the session.

Summary of Intervention Document

- Higher-Self Healing (Problem Strategies, Negative Emotions, Limiting Beliefs)
- Healing with Highest Intention Reframe
- Parts Integration
- Somato-Emotional Drop Down Through
- Forgiveness Exercise
- Goal-setting
- Re-checking Values
- Final Meditation, including meeting the Future You and the Solution Strategy

Chapter 16
Transformational NLP Coaching Techniques

In this chapter we will cover in more detail Transformational NLP coaching techniques, such as Higher-Self Healing for releasing a Problem Strategy, Negative Emotion or a Limiting Belief, Somato-Emotional Drop Down Through, a Forgiveness Exercise, Goal-setting, Final Meditation and writing a letter from the Authentic Self.

First you will be given a script for how to release a Negative Emotion, Problem Strategy or Limiting Belief. You can also do this with a friend, reading the script to each other. Familiarize yourself with the script and then as soon as you can, let go of it and just follow the outline of the process. However, in order for you to let go of the script, you have to know it by heart. (You can download a recorded version of the Higher-Self Healing script from www.nordiclightinstitute.com)

When you use Transformational NLP coaching techniques it is important to remember your outcome at all times. You want to change your thinking and perception of an event in such a way that you are able to let go of the negativity, the illusion of the problem, and instead discover the truth that was always present – the truth that is based in love. Use your process techniques to guide your Unconscious Mind to a place where you are able to connect with your higher, loving wisdom, your own Divine Source, which can then communicate to you the specific Positive Learnings, insights and wisdom you need for healing. *What* this higher, loving wisdom says you cannot know before you do the process, so you have to go through the *experience* of the process. And you have to remember that this higher, loving, divine wisdom is present in each and every one of us – in each and every event we have ever experienced. This means that you can go back to the metaphor of any event and by accessing this higher, loving wisdom, you are able to shine the light of this higher wisdom on the event, so that the perceived negativity disappears and a deep healing takes place.

Higher-Self Healing for releasing a Problem Strategy, Negative Emotion or Limiting Belief

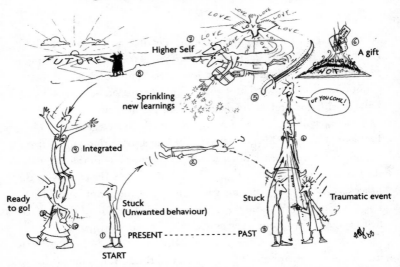

- Timeline – Where is your past? Where is your future? Draw a line between the two. It is only a metaphorical description of your journey through time.
- Find the original event. Ask your Unconscious Mind, "When was the first time you felt this _____ [Problem Strategy, Negative Emotion, Limiting Belief]?"
- Ask your Unconscious Mind to float you up into the air now and allow yourself to go back to that time.
- Float above it and ask for the Positive Learnings/Insights/Wisdom.
- If there are other people at the event, expand your perception. If you need to, do Perceptual Positions (see pages 59–63). Make sure you say everything you have to say, and let the others speak to you, too. Forgive. Cut the cords if needed.

- Light a healing fire and let it cleanse the Negative Emotion away. Then a new positive energy rises up from the fire. Breathe in this positive energy.
- Come back to now, releasing all the _____ (Problem Strategy, Negative Emotion, Limiting Belief), while sprinkling all the Positive Learnings and positive energy into your Timeline all the way back to now.
- Go out to Eternity and meet your Wise Higher Self. Receive your gift from the Chamber of Treasures (see page 81), which will help you on your journey through life.
- See how your future has changed now.

Higher-Self Healing Process

When you do this exercise, you may go to any event in the past, which your Unconscious Mind presents you with in order for you to get the learnings, insights and wisdom you need to release this (Problem Strategy, Negative Emotion or Limiting Belief). It may be from as far back as your childhood, in the womb or even a past life. Just see it as a metaphor your Unconsious Mind feels is the right one for you to work with. It is not the event that is important, but the *Positive Learnings*.

If you do this exercise with a client, just follow the text. The text in square brackets is guidance to the coach. If you do it on your own, imagine you have your Angel Coach sitting on your shoulder, saying:

1. "Ask your Unconscious Mind when was the first time you felt this _____ [Problem Strategy, Negative Emotion, Limiting Belief]? Your Unconscious Mind is very wise and knows about everything that has ever happened to you.

2. "Ask your Unconscious Mind to float you up in the air, all the way back to the first time you felt this _____ [Problem Strategy, Negative Emotion, Limiting Belief], or to the event your Unconscious Mind feels is the right one for you to work with today, so you are able to get the Positive Learnings you need, so you can heal this now. Feel yourself now travel back *into the past*, right down inside the event, or the metaphor, your Unconscious Mind feels is the right one for you to work with.

3. "Then fly up from this event and go to just before the event. Fly high, high up, all the way up to a beautiful, sacred mountain top and sit up here on this beautiful mountain. As you sit up here you notice there is a healing, sacred fire burning up here, like a camp fire. You sit down by this fire, high up here on this mountain and you then look at what is happening down there at that event. What is happening at that event? Now also bring up the version of you that is down there at the event, to be up here with you on this mountain top, so the younger you feels safe up here with you.

4. "[If there are other people at the event. If not, go to Step 6.] If there are other people with you there at the event that you feel are important for you to be able to heal this now, you can now invite them to be up here with you at this sacred mountain top, or you can let them stay down there at the event. Whatever you choose is right for you.

5. "Take the opportunity to speak to each of the other people at the event from the wise part of yourself. First of all, open up the top of your head, draw in a universal white light into your heart and send it to all the others, and also to the younger you. Then let the younger you tell everyone everything this younger you needs to say. You can do this silently in your mind. You create a sacred safe space within you for the younger you to be able to let everything out. Then allow the other people present to reply from their Wise Inner Selves to the younger you, so that they also get to say everything they need to say.

"Then you, as the present-day you, tells everyone everything you need to say, silently in your mind. Let it all out.

"Then allow them to reply from their Wise Inner Selves, so that they can also say to you everything they need to say.

6. "Now send as much love and light as you possibly can to the version of you which was down there at the event, and who is now sitting up here with you on this mountain. Then tell this version of you everything you need to say from the wise part of yourself, and then let this version of you reply to you.

7. "Now also invite your highest, wisest Self to be up here with you. Ask your Wise Higher Self what is the highest intention from this event? What is the highest intention of that? What are the Positive Learnings for you to learn so you can heal this now? What other Positive Learnings are there? [Keep asking for Positive Learnings until you reach a high enough Logical Level of Positive Learnings, so the problem can shift. Write down these learnings after the exercise.]

   "What do you need to know and learn so you can heal this fully now? What do you need to pay attention to so you can do that? What do you need to focus on?

   "Now integrate within you all your insights and learnings.

8. "[If there are other people at the event continue to Step 8. If there are no other people at the event, go to Step 10.] Search your heart to see if you are now ready to tell the other people at this event that you forgive them, or whether there is anything else you need to say first before you can forgive them fully? Know that as you forgive you release yourself from the past. Do that now. Then allow them to do the same to you.

9. "Notice the cords that bind you to the others. Some of these cords may have been formed by negative emotions and negative thoughts. Just notice which of the cords are negative. Then imagine a beautiful golden sword. Take this sword now and cut these negative cords away. First cut them from all around you – front, sides and back – and then cut all around the others, too.

10. "Tell the version of you who was at the event that you forgive him/her and let this version of you say the same to you. Know that forgiveness liberates you completely from the past, so that you are free to create the life you want to live. Now cut any cords and attachments to any negative thoughts and behaviours you may have formed with this old negativity. See a golden sword and cut these cords and attachments now, so that you free yourself from negativity, and also cut through all time and space, freeing you completely from this. Then see again the healing, sacred fire that is burning up here on this mountain top. Place all the cords on this fire and see how the blue-white heat cleanses away all the negative

energies held in these cords until they are all gone. Place on this fire anything else you now want to let go of and see how the fire cleanses it all away, until it is all gone.

11. "Then a new positive energy rises up from the fire, which is a gift to you. Notice what this positive energy, this gift, is. What does it represent for you? Then breathe in this _____ [positive energy], let it fill your lungs fully, and as you breathe out, let it flow to every cell of your being; body, mind and Spirit. Do this once more, please.

12. "Reassure the version of you that was at the event that he/she will never have to experience this again, because you are here now to protect and love him/her. Then take this younger you inside your own heart and allow him/her to grow up into the wise person you are today.

13. "Let this healing fire that is burning up here on this mountain now grow bigger and bigger, until it becomes a huge, powerful column of fire. Then send this healing column of fire down there into the event and let it cleanse and heal the event fully. Let the fire just burn away any old negativity, until all that is left is a beautiful healing light. Then send this column of fire from this event, all the way back to now, and see, feel, hear and notice how it burns away any old negativity – just cleanses it all away, transforms it fully, until all that is left is this beautiful healing light. Then send this column of fire out into your future, allowing it to burn away any obstacles, clearing the path for you, filling your whole future with a healing light, so that you can move with ease into your future. Then let this column of fire come back to this sacred mountain top, where it recedes into being a small healing fire again.

14. "Then float up from this mountain and feel yourself travel back from this event to *now*, and see, feel and notice how you sprinkle all your Positive Insights and Learnings of _____ [your specific Positive Learnings] into your life all the way back to now, like positive seeds that are able to take hold, blossom and enrich your life. In doing this you free yourself from your past, so that you are able to live more fully in the now.

15. "Then travel out into the *future* and see how much it has changed

now, enriched with your new learnings of _____ [your specific Positive Learnings]. Go out one week from now, one month, three months, six months, one year, five years and 10 years, all the way out to eternity. There in eternity you meet your Wise Most Evolved Higher Self. Your Wise Higher Self takes you to a Chamber of Treasures and gives you a gift, a treasure, which will help you on your journey through life. Notice what this gift is. What does this gift represent to you?

16. "Accept this gift and let it now integrate within you. Then travel back to now and let this gift enrich your future all the way back to now. Feel, see and experience how the essence from this gift floats inside every day of your life, all the way from eternity, back to now, and how it helps you to live your life fully, and when you are back in the now, ready to live your life to the full, enriched with your new Positive Learnings _____ [your specific Positive Learnings] and inner gift of _____ [specific gift], then, and only then, can you open your eyes."

Now do the same process with all the Negative Emotions and Limiting Beliefs on your intervention document.

What to do next

Now look at your Intervention Document and do Healing with the Highest Intention Reframe on the problem (see pages 95–101). If you need to also do Parts Integration (see pages 101–6) and after you have done that move onto the next exercise.

Somato-Emotional Drop Down Through

I developed this as a quick way of helping my osteopathic patients release the emotional component of physical pain. It is a mix of various other techniques and has its roots in the NLP technique Drop Down Through. The premise is that we all have a positive inner essence. I will describe a few cases for which I have used the technique in 30-minute osteopathic treatments. Often the process only takes around 10 minutes.

Dealing with sudden onset of insomnia

One man was literally dragged into my osteopathic practice by his wife. He had just lost his job and had been unable to sleep ever since; he complained that his eyes were hurting him during the night. I examined him osteopathically and could feel that he had a highly charged nervous system, causing him to be unable to switch off. While I treated his nervous system osteopathically, I instructed him to float inside his eyes to the area where he would feel the pain, which turned out to be his eyelids. As he floated inside them he first felt anger; it brought up the memory of how his boss had avoided telling him that he was being made redundant, and he felt his boss had been a coward for not talking to him properly. I told him he would be able to go back to this memory later on, and then instructed him to keep dropping through the layers. He eventually came to happiness and strength, which was the level his Unconscious Mind felt he needed to get to. We brought this happiness and strength all the way back up to the anger and he there met his boss again. This time he had the chance to tell his boss everything he needed to say and let his boss reply from his Wise Inner Self. He then could forgive his boss, cut the cords and let it all go.

The result? He could sleep again and he found an even better job within two weeks of his session.

The disappearance of warts

A woman came to see me for a 30-minute appointment. It turned out she had several warts on the soles of her feet, which made it very difficult to walk. She had suffered with them for over 20 years, had been to several consultants and had tried everything, even having them surgically removed, only for them to grow back again. I asked her to float inside the warts and ask them what their highest purpose was for her. "To slow me down," she replied. I then instructed her through a Somato-Emotional Drop Down Through technique, in which she ended up at a beautiful rainbow. The message from the rainbow was for her to enjoy her life. I advised her to meditate on this rainbow every day and take steps to slow down and enjoy her life. The result? Her warts had completely disappeared within a few months.

You can also use this technique on the body area where you felt the emotions associated with the problem. It is a different way into the Unconscious Mind and as you drop through the layers you will be able to release the emotional content held in this problem.

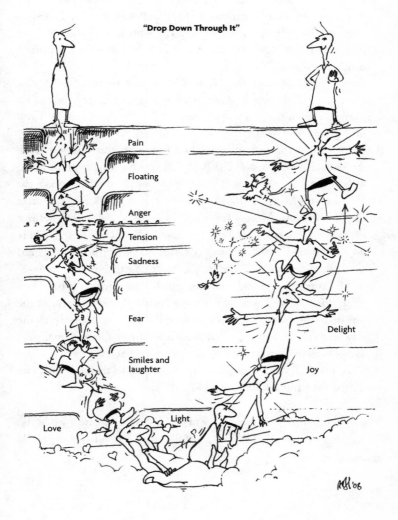

"Drop Down Through It"

Pain

Floating

Anger

Tension

Sadness

Fear

Delight

Smiles and laughter

Joy

Light

Love

Outline of the Process

1. Find the area of the body that is in need of healing, or the body area where you feel your emotions are associated with a particular problem. Float inside it. Notice what it looks like. Sink into it. There will be an emotion there. What is this emotion? Feel it fully – allow it to come up and be expressed. How old were you the first time you experienced this emotion? Is there a memory linked with it? Reassure the younger you that you will soon come back and then continue dropping through.

2. Drop straight through this layer. What is underneath? Feel it fully. Drop straight though it. Keep on dropping and feeling each layer, until you reach the boundary. It feels as if nothing is there, as if you have gone into a void.

3. Drop straight through the boundary, this void. You will now reach the essence within. Go to the Positive Layer the Unconscious Mind feels is the one you need. Then say, "I would now like to ask the Unconscious Mind, is this the level you need to get to?" Calibrate the Unconscious Mind "Yes" and "No" signals. Ask this Positive Essence, "What is it I need to know and learn so I can heal this fully now in my life?", "What do I need to focus on?", "What do I need to pay attention to?", "What are the Positive Learnings here for me?" If this Positive Layer had a colour, which colour would it be? Then bring this Positive Layer, which is the Positive Inner Essence, all the way up to the memory encountered, or, if there is no memory, all the way up to the area in need that you started from. Go to Step 6.

4. Travel back up to the memory. Forgive the others involved.

5. Then bring all the Positive Resources back up to the body area you started with and notice how it looks different now.

The chart opposite gives a summary of the process. Only use it while you are learning the process. Then let go of the chart and follow the process as described above.

Body area
⬇
Negative Layer ➡ How old were you first time you felt this?
Memory linked with it?

⬇
Negative Layer
⬇
Negative Layer
⬇
Negative Layer
⬇
Void
⬇
Positive Layer (You can ask if these had colours, which
colours would they be?
This intensifies the submodalities.)

⬇
Positive Layer ➡ Is this the level you need to get to? Calibrate
"Yes" and "No" signals. If you get a "No" then keep dropping through,
until you get a "Yes". Then bring that essence all the way back up to the
memory encountered, and finally also up to the body area. If a memory
is encountered do the Forgiveness Exercise there.

⬇
Notice that the body area now is positive

Exercise for Somato-Emotional Drop Down Through

(A version can be downloaded from www.nordiclightinstitute.com)

If you do this exercise with a client, just follow the script (remember
to give them time to answer). Text in square brackets is guidance for the
coach. If you do this alone, imagine your Angel Coach is talking to you.

1. "Close your eyes and sink into the stillness within you. Now float
inside your _____ [the body area you are working with]. Really

allow yourself to sink into this area, to be there fully. What does it look like? What does it feel like? There will be an area where this feeling is the most concentrated, where it is the strongest. Float to this area now. Sink into it fully. Allow yourself to really feel this area. Feel it fully. Breathe in the feeling in this area, allow it to come up, allow yourself to really feel it. Embrace it, feel it fully. What is this emotion?

"If you were to know, how old were you the first time you experienced this _____ [named emotion]? Are there any other people connected to this? Is there a memory linked with this? If there is, then promise this younger you that you will come back to him/her later on, in just a few minutes. OK?

2. "Now drop through this emotion to the next layer. What is underneath? [If it is just an emotion, then continue. If you come up with a symbol, such as a stone or fog, just ask your Unconscious Mind what it represents. This usually gives you a feeling, emotion or quality. Then continue.] Allow yourself to really feel it. Breathe it in, embrace it. Feel it fully.

"Now drop straight through it. What is underneath? [If it is a symbol, ask what it represents, so that you get a feeling, an emotion or a quality.] Feel this fully, breathe it in, embrace it and then drop straight through it."

[Keep doing this until there are no more layers and you get to the Void. Some people drop straight through the Void and go from a Negative Layer to a Positive Layer without encountering an obvious Void. That is fine, too.

If you get to the Void let your Angel Coach say,] "This place feels as if there is nothing there. Just allow yourself to drop straight through this Void until you get to the other side [always a Positive Layer]."

[If you don't get a positive layer here, you have not gone through the real Void, but have just encountered some resistance, so just keep *dropping through* the layers until you start to feel you are accessing your inner essence. When you think you are at the right place, let your Angel Coach ask your Unconscious Mind, "Is this the place you need to get to?" Calibrate with your Unconscious Mind "Yes" and "No" signals. If you get a "No" signal, just keep on dropping through. Keep asking the question until you reach the essence you need to get to and confirm that with a "Yes" signal from your Unconscious Mind. If the essence is in the form of a symbol, just ask, "What does this represent for me?"

3. Once you get to the Positive Inner Essence, let your Angel Coach ask you:]

"If this _____ [Inner Essence] had a colour, what colour would it be?

"I also want to ask this _____ [Inner Essence], what is it that it wants you to know and learn so you can heal this fully now in your life? What do you need to pay attention to so you can do that? What do you need to focus on? What are the Positive Learnings it wants you to learn now, so that this can heal fully and completely now?"

4. Let your Angel Coach say the following:

"Now bring this _____ [named Positive Inner Essence and, if you want to, all the other Positive Layers encountered, colour, learnings] all the way back up, back to the area we first started with."

[If you encountered a memory with a younger you, or there were other people connected with this, your Angel Coach says the following (if not, move straight to Step 8):]

"Meet now the Younger You who first experienced this emotion. Hold the Younger You in your arms. Open up the top of your head, draw in a universal white light into your heart and then send this light and love to the Younger You, until he/she sparkles and radiates with this love and light. Then say everything you need to say to each other, so the Younger You can feel loved by you and safe again. Ask the Younger You if there is anyone else he/she needs to talk to so that this can heal fully now." [If there is, then do Step 5. Otherwise go to Step 7.]

5. "Invite them [the others] to be here with you now. Ask them if it is OK with them to let you heal this fully now. Get a sense of whether they say "Yes" and then turn to the person the Younger You feels is most involved in this. Imagine the top of your head opening up and letting Universal White Light and Love Energy flow through you into your heart and out to the Younger You. Then imagine the

Younger You, being filled with this light, sends some of this light out to _____ [named other person]. Then let the Younger You say everything that needs to be said to this person, and then let the Present-Day You say to _____ [named other person] everything you need to say from the wise part of you now. Let it all out.

"When you feel you have completely said everything you need to say from your heart and soul, then allow _____ [named other person] to also say to the Younger You and to the Present-Day You everything they need to say from their Wise Self. Continue doing this until you all have said everything you need to say.

"Are you, and the Younger You, now ready to say to the other person that you forgive them, knowing that as you forgive you free yourself from the past, because forgiveness is a gift you give yourself? Then say to each other that you forgive each other.

[If there is someone else the Younger You needs to do this process with, then do Step 5 again. Only move to Step 6 once this is completed.]

6. "Now notice the cords that bind you together. Some of these cords might be negative. Now cut any negative cords with a beautiful golden sword. First cut them from your end and then from the other person's end.

"Now visualize a healing fire, place these cords on this fire and see how the fire cleanses all the negative emotions and energies held in these cords away, until they have all gone. Then place all your Negative Emotions on this fire and see how the fire purifies and cleanses them too, until they have all gone. Then slowly, a new positive energy is rising from the fire, which is a gift to you and which will help you on your journey through life. Notice what this positive energy is and then breathe it in. Let it fill your lungs fully and as you breathe out let this _____ [positive energy] flow to every cell of your being: body, mind and Spirit and especially to the area of your body where you first started this process.

7. "Tell the Younger You that you are here now to love, protect and guide him/her. Take the Younger You inside yourself and allow this younger version of you to grow up into the wise person you are today.

8. "Now invite your wise Higher Self to be here with you and ask what the Positive Learnings are here for you, so you can heal this fully now. Make sure you get these learnings.

9. "Then fill your _____ [body area you started with when doing this exercise, such as heart or stomach] with your _____ [Positive Layers, Learnings, Positive Colour and Essence given] and allow it to heal this area fully now. Notice what your _____ [body area] looks like now. [It should now look and feel positive.]

10. "Imagine you go out into the future now and fill your whole future with these _____ [Positive Learnings, Colours, Positive Essence and Insights]. Go out one week from now, one month, three months, one year, five years, 10 years, go all the way out to eternity and fill your whole future with these Positive Learnings, Colours and Positive Emotions. There in eternity you meet your most evolved Higher Self, who takes you to the Chamber of Treasures, where they give you a gift, which will help you with all of this. What is the gift you receive? What does it represent for you? How will it help you? Accept this gift now and thank your Higher Self for being in your life. Then take this gift and let the essence from this gift flow into every day of your life, all the way from eternity back to now, and then let it integrate fully within you in the here and now.

11. "Then rest in your inner stillness for a few moments, and when you feel ready to act upon all your insights and learnings, ready to live your life to the full, then, and only then, you can open your eyes."

The Gift of Forgiveness

I would urge you to really practise forgiveness in your own life. Forgiveness sounds easy, but it is harder to do in reality. However, it is the most important ingredient in healing yourself.

The importance of forgiveness

When you forgive you release yourself from the bondage of the past and this frees you to live fully in the now, enjoying your life.

Then why is it so difficult for us to forgive? That's because we are hurting and often we want the person responsible to know we are hurting. Or we want them to admit that they were wrong and that we are justified in feeling angry, upset or hurt. Therefore we refuse to forgive people we consider to have hurt us in some way and instead hold on to past hurts, because we fear that if we forgive them, we let them off the hook, and acknowledge that they were right and that we have somehow lost an imaginary battle. Instead we walk around carrying the burden of our past heavily on our shoulders, and hold on firmly to our Negative Thoughts and Emotions. Anyone who has ever been really angry with another person knows how this starts to eat away at your inner life.

Let the past go. Just let it go. You do that by releasing the Negative Emotions, Limiting Beliefs and Limiting Decisions and instead choosing to view each event from a wise, compassionate and positive perspective, and then you need to forgive everyone involved, including yourself.

This frees your mind from the past. It is such a miracle when you do forgive someone, because you feel as if you have been freed from a prison. Whereas when you are angry with someone, you keep thinking about them. Often they pop into your head on a daily basis, sometimes several times a day. Once you have forgiven and let go, you stop thinking about them. You have given your mind the antidote to a bitter and negative poison. This is your true gift to yourself, so please realize that you forgive someone in order for *you* to be happy and not to let the other person off the hook. You actually let yourself off the hook because you hooked these Negative Thoughts onto yourself. Once you fully understand this it becomes so much easier to forgive, because you realize that it is truly the only wise choice to make, because this choice will lead you to your own inner peaceful Heaven.

If someone has abused you in the past or done something terrible to you, and you now feel your happiness and peace of mind is dependent on whether they apologize or not, then stop. Do not give your power away in this way, by letting your happiness depend on what someone else does. Or perhaps you always craved acknowledgment from a specific person in your life, but you never got it. Perhaps you went to extremes and you still never felt acknowledged. Then stop! Take your power back and instead start to appreciate and acknowledge yourself.

Forgiveness Exercise

This is a very powerful exercise (adapted from the Ho'oponopono of Hawaiian Huna), which only takes 5–10 minutes and helps you to start a deep process of forgiveness. It is also great to do in relation to those you love deeply and whom you just feel you want to connect with in a more loving way (so no need to forgive). I will outline it for you here, so you can easily do this exercise at any time. Please practise it in relation to all those you have listed on your Intervention Document. As a rough guide I would suggest you do it in relation to your parents, siblings, partner and children, as applicable, and in that order. Text in square brackets is to help you find your way around the steps more easily.

(A version is available to download at www.nordiclightinstitute.com)

1. Close your eyes and see this person in front of you. Ask this person (silently in your mind) if it is OK for you to heal your relationship with them. Get a sense of whether they give you permission. (Most people do, but if they don't you have to respect that and not do this exercise in relation to them.) Then you can go ahead and do this process.

2. Imagine now that you open up the top of your head, draw in universal white light into your heart and keep sending this person this love and light until you see them sparkle with light.

3. Then tell them everything you need to tell them. Let it all out. You can do this silently in your mind.

4. Now allow the other person to respond from their Wise Inner Self. You can let them do this silently in your mind.

5. Ask your Wise Higher Self, "What are the Positive Learnings here for me to learn? What other Positive Learnings are there?"

6. Search deep within your heart to see if you are willing to completely forgive this person now, knowing that as you forgive, you release yourself from this pain you felt in the past. Then tell this person you forgive them and that you now let this go.

7. Allow this person to say to you, too, that they also forgive you, or that they are sorry if they have caused you any pain.

8. Then either take this person inside your heart or cut the cords that bind you together. [If you take this person inside your heart then move straight down to Step 11.]

9. If you cut the cords, you cut the projection that you have of this person, which allows you to see this person for how they are now and not the way they were in the past. [If you want to cut the cords continue with the exercise. Otherwise go straight to Step 11.]

10. Notice if there are any cords that bind you together and now imagine a golden sword and cut the cords first from your end and then from the other person's end. Then place these cords on a healing, sacred fire and see how the blue-white heat of the fire cleanses away all the negative energies held in these cords, until they are all gone. Then a new positive energy rises from the fire, which is a gift to you. Breathe this positive energy in. Let it fill your lungs, and as you breathe out let it flow to every cell of your being; body, mind and Spirit.

11. Now ask your Wise Higher Self, "What is it you want me to learn so that I can move forward in my life aligned with my Spirit?" "What is it this person is teaching me by being in my life?" Trust the answers you receive.

12. Then thank this person for allowing you to do this healing work.

When you do this process you start to realize that everyone in your life has something positive to teach you about yourself and your path. This allows you to let go of your resentment, hurt and need for others to be the way you want them to be. It also helps you to become compassionate and grateful for all the lessons other people are helping you to learn, and you start to realize that no one in your life comes along by accident, but that they are drawn to you and you to them, so that you can both learn, heal and grow. Sometimes that healing and growing is nice and smooth; at other times it is painful and messy. It is similar to when a baby is born; it is a very painful, difficult and bloody experience, for both the baby and the mother, but they have to go through it, in order for both of them to enjoy being together and help each other learn more about love, themselves and the world. If they were, instead, so focused on the pain of the birth that they avoided going through with it, then they would miss all the wonderful opportunities life has to bring them.

Being honest with yourself and forgiving of yourself and others is very much the same as giving birth, because what you are really doing is giving birth to yourself – your true, authentic self, your spiritual self, your loving, most resourceful, self. The self that has chosen to live in your particular body, at this particular time, has chosen the people you have in your life in order for you to grow, and has set out certain things it wants you to learn and grow from in this life. But you can only do that when you start taking responsibility for yourself, your thoughts and your actions, letting go of the past, forgiving yourself and others, and start being loving, compassionate and honest. When you start living your life literally from the heart, you allow yourself to live in balance with the physical, emotional, mental and spiritual aspects of yourself, because your heart is the gate-keeper to all these worlds.

"Inner peace can be reached only when we practise forgiveness. Forgiveness is the letting go of the past, and it is therefore the means for correcting our misperceptions."
> Gerald G. Jampolsky, *Love is Letting Go of Fear*

Goal-setting

Goal-setting is really important, because it shows your Unconscious Mind what it is you want, and it also allows you to become clear within yourself about where you are going and what you need to do to achieve that. During a Transformational Break-Through Healing Session make sure you set at least three goals and ideally also set more goals after the session.

Set your goals from your heart, *not* your ego

Unfortunately there are many books and courses telling you to set goals so that you can acquire more "stuff": more money, a bigger house, more power and so on. This is setting goals from your ego, which believes that you can only be happy and satisfied when you have more stuff. Instead set goals from your heart; from that passion and longing that lives there. If you feel a longing inside your heart that you want to live closer to Nature and have more living space, then set a goal about that. If, however, you want to live in a bigger house because you want to impress your friends and neighbours, then that goal comes from your ego – so please do not set it. It will just bring frustration, emptiness and sadness.

Your goal also has to be "smart". You may know about "smart" goals, but the way I outline it here is probably a bit different, as I give a more esoteric slant to it. What SMART means is:

S – Simple and specific

M – Measurable and meaningful

A – Achievable, as if now (you set it in the present tense, as if it is happening now), in all areas of life

R – Realistic and responsible

T – Toward what you want and when you want it ("timed") – meaning that you have a deadline for when you want to have achieved it.

It is important that the goal is *specific*, because the more specific it is, the easier it is for the Unconscious Mind to know what it is you really want. It has to be *simple* so that it is easy for the Unconscious Mind to understand fully what it is you want. However, a specific and simple goal can be a goal such as, "I am happy", or "I am filled with energy and enthusiasm about my life". Even though you are not specifying exactly how you are happy, you are specifying the emotion you want, a way of being, and from that emotion and way of being stems a certain thought pattern, something your Unconscious Mind is very aware of, so it will help you by producing your inner unconscious programming of being happy, and being filled with enthusiasm and energy about your life. It is always best to set goals about positive ways of *being*, as from your positive being flows right action. This often produces more positive results than setting goals about *having*, such as, "I have happiness", because before you have happiness you have to *be* happiness. The quickest way of having happiness is being happy and being the source of happiness for someone else. This is true of everything. If you want to *have* abundance, then be abundant and be the source of abundance for someone else. Abundance will flow to you also from the outside world and before you know it you will have abundance. You have immense abundance within you, just waiting for you to tap into it. You have an abundance of love, happiness, warmth, empathy, affection and wisdom within you. Abundance is not only about money. Abundance is a state of being. If you want to have more money in your life, then be abundant and be the source of abundance for someone else. *Give to others*, and *be willing to receive* from others.

A goal also has to be *measurable* so you know exactly what it is you want and if it is *meaningful* to you then you are going to have the drive necessary to take all the steps needed in order for you to achieve your goal.

It has to be *achievable*, because if it is not then your Unconscious Mind is not going to try to achieve it for you. Remember, though, that the Unconscious Mind has an enormous amount of wisdom, Positive Resources and intelligence within it, so we are all able to create true miracles in our lives. Think outside the box, so free your mind from any restraints and aim for the stars. Remember, everything once started off as a thought, so aim as high as you can with your thoughts and keep raising the bar.

"As if now" (as if it is happening right now) is the most important part, because when you state "as if now", your Unconscious Mind acts upon it immediately.

"All areas of life" means that what you want has to enhance your life overall. For example, if you have a goal of moving to Australia, but you also have a goal of finishing your studies, then these two goals will be in conflict with each other.

"Realistic" is important, because if your goal is not realistic then your Unconscious Mind is not going to try to achieve it for you. For example, if you are a world-class 100-metre-sprint athlete then it is realistic to set a goal to win the Olympics in your particular sport, but if you never exercise and haven't got the body of an athlete, then it may not be realistic to set a goal to win the Olympic gold medal in the 100-metre sprint. "Responsible" means that the full responsibility of achieving this goal lies completely with you.

"Toward what you want" is vital, because you get what you focus on. So make sure none of your goals is stated in the negative and about what you do not want. "Timed" is important because it gives the Unconscious Mind a direction about when you want to have achieved this goal. I tend to time the goal after I start the goal-setting exercise, so as to make sure I time it with my Unconscious Mind, instead of my Conscious Mind. You will see what I mean later on in this chapter (see pages 215–216).

Never state a goal about a person other than yourself. All your goals should be just about you, because if you force your will upon another person you are not being "ecological" (ethical, in alignment with your Higher Self and the Higher Divine Will), because the other person may not want this goal you have set for them. You can state a goal that you are happy in your relationship with someone, but you cannot state a goal that they are happy with you. That is up to them, not you. Instead of saying "My partner and I are now living in a happy, loving relationship", you would say "I am loving and happy in my relationship with my partner". This is the difference between "black" magic (forcing your will upon another) and "white" magic (working for the higher good of everyone and never imposing your will upon anyone else).

You also need to make sure that your goals will not affect someone else negatively, such as if you want to buy a specific house, you should not request a goal about a particular house, because perhaps the people already living in it want to continue living there, or the house is meant for someone else. Instead, set a goal about all the specific qualities you want your house to have, such as five bedrooms, big garden, a study and in the catchment area of a good school. Then leave it up to your Unconscious Mind and the Universe to attract to you the perfect house for you, instead of you narrowing down the possibility by focusing on just one particular house.

The importance of linguistics

Never state your goals in the negative (you get what you focus on, so you would attract that which you do not want more to you) – for example, "I am *not* poor", "I am *not* unhappy" or "I am *not* a failure". Instead say, "I am abundant", "I am happy", "I am a success".

Also avoid saying, "I want", such as in, "I *want* to be abundant", because you get the wanting of it; that is you never become abundant –

all you get is the *wanting* of wanting to be abundant. Instead say, "I am abundant" or "I am living an abundant life".

Never use "I will", such as in, "I *will* be happy". This is because "will" implies the future, so you never get it – it is always in the future. Instead say, "I am happy".

Make sure your goal is stated in the present tense – for example, "I am healthy and happy".

Preparing for the goal-setting exercise

Before you set a goal ask yourself, "For what purpose do I want this goal?" When you know the purpose for wanting something, it gives you that extra drive that will make sure you do everything you need to do to get you the results you want.

Then you ask yourself, "What is my highest intention behind wanting this goal?"

When your intention is coming from a place of love, you are much more likely to be able to manifest it in a happy, fulfilling way.

Goal-setting exercise

Now take your first goal and imagine your Angel Coach asking your Unconscious Mind, "What is the last step that has to happen for you to know that you have achieved it?" (Formulate this step and write it down on a chart like the one shown on page 216.)

Now close your eyes and visualize this last step. Make it the most real and intense for you. Then step out of the picture so that you see yourself in it, as if you are looking at a photo or movie of yourself. Blow four deep breaths into it as this will help to energize your goal with your Life Energy. Take the picture and float above it and ask your Unconscious Mind when you would like to have achieved this goal. Then take the picture and float all the way out into the future, and at the appropriate time let go of the picture and see it float down inside your future. Then notice how all the events from then to now realign themselves to support your goal. Then say to yourself, "This, or something better, now manifests for me for the highest good of all concerned." Now carry out the same process with all the other goals.

Goal	Last step	Date
_____	_____	_____
_____	_____	_____
_____	_____	_____
_____	_____	_____
_____	_____	_____
_____	_____	_____

Re-checking values

Now re-check values, making sure that they are all 100 per cent positive.

What your Angel Coach says when you re-check values

"OK, we are now going to re-check your values. As we have done all this work together and you have had all your wonderful Positive Learnings, Insights and Wisdom communicated to you from your Unconscious Mind, your inner screening system will have completely changed. Remember how your inner screening system was made up of your beliefs, values and past experiences? As we have now released all those old Negative Beliefs and have healed how you experience your past, your inner screening system will have changed and you should be left with all your values 100 per cent positive. I can only let you go on to finish this work once all these values are 100 per cent positive, as you need to have changed your *thinking*, so that it is absolutely positive. Then it is up to you to take action and that is your responsibility. My responsibility is to make sure your *thinking* has changed, as you are sitting here with me, now."

"What is important to you now about _____ [relationships, family, work, health, personal or spiritual development – whichever area you elicited the values in before the intervention]?"

"What else is important to you now about _____ [X area]?"

Keep asking this until you have a list of values – at least eight to 10 values.

Then number them in order of importance, with "one" meaning "most important" and "eight" meaning "least important". You can do this by asking yourself, "If you could only have one, which one would it be? If you could only have two?" And so on.

Once you have them in order, your Angel Coach asks: "Why is value _____ [specific value] important to you? [Ideally now state a positive reason, giving you a positive Internal Representation.] As you think about that now, how much positive energy do you feel about this?"

If you have done all the work in the Break-Through Healing Session you will say "100 per cent", because once you have released all the negativity held in your old "problem" you will be left with 100 per cent pure positive energy. Most people actually say 100 per cent here.

If you do not say 100 per cent positive, your Angel Coach then says, "OK, as you are now, in your thoughts, is there anything that could be stopping you from having 100 per cent positive energy moving toward creating _____ [specific value] in this area of your life?"

Usually most people say, "No". Your Angel Coach then says, "Great, so how much positive energy, as you are in your thoughts right now, do you feel in relation to _____ [specific value] now, enabling you to move toward positively creating _____ [specific value] in the future?" People usually say 100 per cent here.

Look at your values now and check to see whether they all have 100 per cent positive energy, as your *thinking* now will have changed dramatically, thanks to you having done all this work on yourself.

Remember, too, that it is now up to you to actually follow all the Positive Learnings, Insights and Wisdom your Unconscious Mind and Higher Self have communicated to you, so if that old doubt creeps into your mind, just remember that doubt will only be satisfied when it has *proof* that you have changed, and it can only have proof with *time*. So just say to the doubt, "Hello, my friend. Just come with me into the future and you will see that in three months' time, or six months, or perhaps even sooner than that, as we look back on today, you will see that I have indeed changed, because I now have had the chance to live out and act upon all these amazing insights, wisdom and learnings my Unconscious Mind and Wise Higher Self have communicated to me. And, I promise you, I will, from now on, act upon these insights." Now, doubt being doubt, it will still doubt you, but you know better. And then, with time, you will, indeed, look back upon today and realize, "Wow, I did it! I did change! Amazing!" And then doubt will rest for a while, only later to find something else to doubt. There is no point in arguing with doubt. It's best just not pay much attention to it.

Final Meditation

In the Final Meditation I want you to relax fully, connecting with the peace and stillness within you and I also want you to feed back your own Solution Strategy, as well as all the major Positive Learnings your Unconscious Mind and Higher Self have communicated to you during the session. So look at your Solution Strategy now and write down all your major Positive Learnings, so that you remember them clearly.

Write them down here:

Solution Strategy

_____

_____

_____

Major Positive Learnings and Insights

_____

_____

_____

_____

_____

_____

Once you have done that, listen to the Final Meditation track on the version that you can download from www.nordiclightinstitute.com Remember the message from your Future You and write it down here:

_____

_____

_____

_____

Then here write the letter from your authentic self (do that after you have listened to the downloadable version).

Letter from my Authentic Self

_____

_____

_____

_____

_____

_____

_____

_____

_____

_____

_____

_____

_____

_____

_____

_____

Summary

Well done for taking yourself through the deeply healing and transformative Break-Through Healing Session. Know that you can carry out this process any time you encounter a problem. I take myself through this process regularly, as I want to be able to let go of my different layers of negativity, so that I am more able to connect to my inner wisdom, light and spiritual guidance. So make a commitment to work on yourself personally and spiritually. You will be rewarded a thousand-fold.

Transformational NLP uses exquisite tools for facilitating deep healing and the more evolved you are, the more able you will be to create the life you want to lead. The more you work on yourself, the more spiritual energy, light and wisdom you will have available within you, for you to use in manifesting your most fulfilling life – ever. It is also important to remember that working on ourselves is a journey – and a process – so we have to refrain from thinking that we are ever finished. There is always more to learn, more discoveries to be made, another layer to shed, another level of wisdom to evolve to.

So be courageous! Be daring! Explore the wonderful adventure that awaits you, as you dive deep into the depths of your mind, soul and Spirit. You have within you untold riches, fantastic resources, exquisite wisdom and you find all of these things when you journey into your Inner Self and connect with your Divine Self. And that is such a journey!

Thank you for doing this work with me and I wish you all the happiness, love, wisdom, fulfilment and divine inspiration from the bottom of my heart and soul.

Cissi Williams, Sigtuna, Sweden

PART 6

Additional Information for Coaches

Chapter 17
Important Pointers

Before you work with someone

Here are some important considerations before you start working with someone. As a general rule, never work with a client who has a problem you are dealing with yourself (and have not overcome yet). For example, if you are dealing with relationships issues, then do not work with a client who is dealing with exactly the same issue. If you stop yourself following your dreams because you worry about money, then do not coach a client who has the same problem. If you hate your ex-partner and have not been able to forgive him or her, then do not coach a client who wants to forgive an ex-partner. If you do work with someone who is going through the same issues, then you will not be able to pace and lead them out of the problem, and even if your client gets a successful result and many Positive Learnings, the chances are you will end up "stealing" positive energy from your client and this is not ethical.

However, once you have overcome an issue yourself, then you are in a *great* position to coach others in the same context, because you *know* it is possible to solve it. Of course, you can coach clients within contexts where you have never had a problem, just not within the contexts where you are still having problems yourself!

When not to help someone

It is important to know when not to help someone. In the first instance, do not help someone who does not want to be helped and I would strongly urge you to *stay away from friends and family*. Let them be and if they need help then send them to a different therapist. Why? Because you will ruin the basis of your relationship, so that you become their therapist and they might not feel comfortable with you delving into their psyche. In addition, they might not be able to be completely honest with you, as some of their "stuff" might be linked to you or to people you know. Above all, it will be difficult for you to be completely objective – and being objective is the same as being able to hold up a mirror for the person you are working with, so that they can see their reflection. If you are not being clear yourself, you will be holding up a distorted mirror, and that is a big "no, no" when using NLP as a tool for healing with the spirit.

The need to work on yourself

If you want to be able to work with others, you have to "walk your talk". You have to still your mind regularly through meditation, or carrying out an activity that helps to stop that inner monkey brain; get your own life in order; be compassionate with yourself; and look at all your own "stuff" – your own Limiting Behaviours and Negative Thought patterns – and take steps to release them.

When you work with someone

The importance of developing wisdom

A really important point is that, the more you practise these techniques, linguistics and tools, the more effective you will become in using them. What is also important is that the more you have developed yourself personally and spiritually, the more wisdom you have within, and it is this wisdom that *directs* how, when and with whom you use the variety of skills, linguistics, techniques and tools, and it is also this wisdom that intuitively *guides* you to play with all the linguistics, skills, tools and techniques, so that you end up with something unique for each client.

My main advice is that you always trust this inner wisdom to guide you and that you should always look for the Higher Logical Level. So ask yourself internally, "What is it this person has not noticed, which if they did notice, the solution would start to reveal itself?"

Then guide your questioning in such a way as to enable the client to find the solutions within themselves. You want to empower your client and the way you do this is to take them through processes where they connect more fully with who they truly are. That means discovering their own inner Positive Learnings, Insights, Wisdom and Resources – not for you to tell them the solution.

The importance of letting go of the need to be liked

When you work with someone you have to let go of your need to be liked, respected and understood. Clients do not come to you to like you. They come because they want to heal and to become who they truly are. That means you cannot play along with the little "games" they play – such as playing helpless, confused, angry, depressed, blaming, sad or whatever negative behaviour they are displaying. You know that this behaviour, this "game", is not who they truly are, and if you were to react to their "game-playing", by getting angry yourself, giving them sympathy, or being more nice to them by giving them extra attention, then you would be feeding this behaviour.

For example, if I have a student who gets very angry every time she is challenged, would I be helping her if I backed off or tried to be extra nice to her? No, I would not. So I point out to her that this behaviour is her own creation and that she has to deal with it. It has nothing to do with me. I also know that this is not the first time she has used anger as a way of trying to control others.

If I have a client who gets confused every time we get close to uncovering what is really causing the problem, would I be assisting him if I believed the confusion was real? No, I would not. I know the confusion is just a smoke screen, giving my client a way out of actually having to deal with the real issues and thereby taking responsibility for them.

What about when someone gets really anxious and panicky? Should I not be extra nice to them? Absolutely not! Being extra nice to people who display anxiety and panic would be giving extra fuel to this behaviour, and the chances are that they are already doing that in their lives. A woman I saw to help her with panic attacks would get them every time she drove faster than 50 miles per hour or whenever she drove over a bridge. Initially she would get them when she drove over a really high bridge and so she then stopped the car and her husband took over the driving. Then the same thing happened over a small bridge; again they stopped the car and her husband took over. Then she could not drive even over a tiny canal bridge. Following this, it also started happening on motorways, so again they stopped the car and her husband took over the driving. Then it happened on roads faster than 70 miles per hour and again her husband took over. Then it was faster than 50 miles per hour. My client was by now virtually unable to drive, as most routes contained some roads faster than 50 miles per hour and crossed some bridges.

Then she started to get panicky every time she had to go higher than the third floor in a building, regardless of whether she had walked up the stairs, taken a lift or gone up an escalator. It was a real problem because she worked on the fourth floor of her office building. Her manager found space for her on the third floor. However, after some months this, too, created anxiety and panic, so they moved her to the second floor. But even that had now started to cause problems. Her boss finally got to the end of his tether, which was why she came to see me in the first place.

When we went back to the very first time she experienced this problem she was a small child on holiday with her parents and they were going to stay in a hotel that had a lift. My client, then aged only eight, became terrified of the lift, and her mother agreed to take the stairs – six floors up! Because the eight-year-old got tired legs, her mother carried her. This fed my client's belief and anxiety that somehow lifts were dangerous. It also gave her extra attention and this was the first time she realized that by being anxious she could get others to bail her out of having to deal with difficult situations. Did she experience anxiety and panic when she was going through a Break-Through session with me? Of course she did. I completely ignored it, tapped her on her hands and told her, "Stop that … now! Just let it go! You have done it for long enough and enough is enough. You are so much more than that old behaviour." And I just continued with whatever we were doing.

During my sessions and trainings, I often tap people (gently "smack" them on their hands or legs) when they go into a behaviour that is not serving them. I pre-frame it beforehand, so they are warned that this is something I do when they go into a behaviour that weakens them.

When to give sympathy and when not to

I also teach my students when *not* to touch someone in a sympathetic way, or give them extra sympathetic attention – and that is when someone is addicted to the drama of their emotions. Giving sympathy will cause them to be more stuck in the drama. The client is so used to getting attention for all the drama she has created in her life that giving her more attention when she does this in a session is just feeding this behaviour. When someone is addicted to the drama, my intention is to help her learn that she can, indeed, let go of her negative emotions quickly. Often she has a belief that she can only let the emotions go if she first goes into them and really, really feels them – staying in there for ages. Then she can start to let them go, usually with someone else's help, so she ends up receiving a great deal of attention during the process. This makes for a very slow process and is something that this person will have done many times in her life.

I work very differently with someone who has difficulty feeling and expressing her emotions – then I do give her more time and attention. I may encouragingly touch her arm and say to her, "You are doing really well", while still continuing to take her through the process. If I were to try to speed her up, as in the example above, I would not be helping her, because she has probably often used her mind to shut herself off from her emotions and it is now key to let her *experience* the emotions and then let them go. Often this type of client has an easier time letting the emotions go, because they are not addicted to them, while the first type is often addicted to their negative emotions, and the attention this gives them from others.

Now I know that the truth about the people I am working with is that they are so much more than the behaviour they are displaying, and by not being fooled by the behaviour I am able to guide them out of it – if they choose to let me do this.

Traumatic experiences

What about when people have been through really traumatic experiences in their lives? Should we not give them extra sympathy then? Well, no. Sympathy will not help them, as that is "feeling sorry" for them. Be compassionate, but not sympathetic. Whatever happened took place in the past and it is only creating a problem now because they still hold onto it in their mind. By remembering that the person has all the resources to solve this, and by guiding them to find the learnings and insights needed to let the past go, you are helping to transform their life – so that they are free from the past. If you were to give the client sympathy, you might be feeding the need for them to get attention for what happened to them in the past, and this can cause them to remain stuck there. So never give sympathy, only empathy and compassion. Compassion, by the way, is not a gentle force, as many believe. It is a very strong force, where you see the truth in someone – and you communicate that truth.

Knowing the linguistics

You have to know the linguistics and the techniques inside out before you embark on taking someone through a Transformational Break-Through Healing Session, and you need to be a qualified Master Practitioner of NLP before you take a client through this process. I feel it is a great responsibility taking someone on this journey, so make sure you have done the Break-Through Healing Session yourself many, many times before you take someone else through it.

Detaching yourself from the drama

Remember, when you do take yourself through these techniques, that everything you are experiencing is just in your head, so *it is not real*. It is an illusion. What is real is that you are safe, going on a journey inside your own mind. You truly need to understand this if you are going to be able to take someone else through this journey. If you allow yourself to get panicky when taking yourself through these exercises, and you are training to be a coach, then you need to do much more work on yourself before you take someone else through it. You truly have to understand, deep within, that it is all an illusion; it is all in your head, and when you allow yourself to become scared by what you are imagining in your mind, you are buying into the drama of that illusion. What took place happened a long time ago. It is not real! What is real is that you are sitting somewhere going on an imaginary journey in your mind.

Buying into the drama is what clients have done, isn't it? So how can you pace and lead them out of that drama, if you have not detached yourself from it?

Logical Levels

Use Logical Levels when you are working on someone. This means you are able to read beneath what the person is saying, as well as seeing the Higher Logical Level of what is really going on. You direct your questioning from this higher awareness. You want to be able to identify the metaphor of how they have been able to create this problem in the first place. You will find this metaphor in their past by using your questioning techniques. You want to be able to see a pattern emerge.

Correct diagnosis

Just as when you go and see an osteopath, doctor or dentist, you want them to carry out a thorough examination so that they are able to diagnose what is going on, you as a coach have to do the same. You do this during your questioning session. You use your Break-Through questions as a red thread – like the spinal column – and then you shoot off from each question using your linguistics, in order to diagnose the structure of the problem. You may end up diagnosing several Problem Strategies, Parts Conflicts, body parts for where to do a Drop Down Through, and several Limiting Beliefs and Negative Emotions. As you diagnose these make a note of them (I use different coloured pens to make this easier), and then after your questioning you will transfer all of this to an Intervention Document.

The deeper you can go into the client's Unconscious Mind with your questioning, and the more correct your diagnosis is, the more profound the intervention techniques will be.

The second metaphor

It is important to find the first metaphor during your *questioning*, so that you can see a pattern emerging from something that has happened in the past, and how that has caused the client to create the problem they are experiencing now.

You receive the second metaphor during the *intervention*, and you will usually find it when doing Higher Self Healing to release a Problem Strategy, Limiting Belief or Negative Emotion. You discover it by finding an event, which contains the perfect metaphor of the actual problem.

Remember, it is just a metaphor, so it can be any event or metaphor that provides the perfect setting for the client to get the Positive Learnings needed to shift and heal the "problem". The point is that you know you have found it because it perfectly mirrors the presenting problem.

Some examples

A woman I saw felt she was selfish, greedy and a generally unpleasant person. She also had a problem with overeating. When we went back to the root cause, she returned to a time in the womb when she realized that she was not the only one in the womb – her twin sister was there, too. She panicked, thinking there would not be enough nourishment to support both of them, so she started trying to get most of the "food". This resulted in her being twice the weight of her sister at birth and she formed an inner belief that she was selfish, greedy and unpleasant – a perfect metaphor of the presenting problem.

Another client believed she could never get what she wanted, while others always could – especially her sister. As she went back to the root cause she floated to an event where she and her sister were given new clothes. My client received practical boyish-looking clothes, while her sister received pretty girlish clothes, even though my client also wanted to have pretty clothes. She then formed a belief that she could never have what she wanted; a perfect metaphor of the presenting problem.

When you, as a coach, realize you have come across a perfect metaphor of the presenting problem, it is *vital* that you help to facilitate your client to get really high-level Positive Learnings and Insights, because it will be these that will help to change the thought patterns, perceptions and beliefs necessary to facilitate deep inner healing. So the Positive Learnings have to be of a high enough Logical Level of *healing*, in order to fully shift and heal the problem.

Process and content

It is important to know the distinction between process and content. As a practitioner you leave the content to the client, while you use all the processes and tools effectively. You can, of course, use the words your client gives you – just make sure you use the exact words the client does, so you avoid putting your own content in. This also means that, for example, if what your client is saying does not make sense to you, or is not grammatically correct – *do not change it*. I have witnessed coaches starting to change what their client is saying just because it was not grammatically correct, or because by changing it, it made more sense to them. *Never, ever do this.* You want to help your client, and the way to do that is to use the *exact structure* of the linguistics your client gives you.

Once you have developed some knowledge and acquired wisdom, you may at times offer advice and suggestions to your clients. However, I would urge you not to do this until you are highly experienced. The simple reasons being:

- You might be completely wrong and give advice and suggestions that are not helpful to the client.
- Even if your suggestions are helpful, they may cause the client to try to become dependent on you, thereby weakening their own ability to find their own inner answers.
- As soon as you start giving advice you might start to become prey to your own inner ego – the ego that thinks you are better, smarter, more evolved, more enlightened than others. This is a real trap and in order to avoid falling into this trap, you must refrain from giving advice and instead guide your questioning so that your clients find their own answers.
- Many clients have a tendency to want to try to put those in authority on a pedestal, and when you give advice you can easily end up on one. You can then also start to believe you belong up there. There is only one place to go from a pedestal – and that is down. Never, ever believe you are more, or better, than others. We are all one – on the same level. Also never believe you are a lesser person than others. We all have equal value.

If you do give advice:

- Just give general recommendations, such as, "Meditation is good for you", "Follow your heart", "Trust your intuition", "Practise seeing the positive in every situation" and so on. And, of course, use any of the Positive Learnings and Insights your client's own Unconscious Mind and Higher Self have communicated during the session.

Avoid giving advice such as:

- I think you should leave your husband.
- Why don't you tell your boss what a complete fool he is?
- What I would do in your situation is quit my job.
- You probably have been sexually abused in the past – it's just that you don't remember it.
- You can never forgive your mother for doing that. Just accept that you cannot forgive her.

I know these seem absurd, but I have heard these pieces of advice being given by coaches and therapists to their clients. This is, of course, content imposition at its worst. *Never, ever do this.*

Creating a sacred space for clients

How do you create a sacred emotional space for healing, a space where the client feels as if you care, as if you truly understand them?

The answer is, you need to listen, listen and listen. Truly listen, without judging and with great rapport. If you were in your client's shoes how would you think? You don't have to agree with people to accept them as a person. You can respect their opinions and completely disagree with them. You can show empathy without having to agree or compromise your beliefs or integrity.

I often see clients who are very different from myself, with different values, beliefs, thoughts and behaviours. In the session I completely empty myself of any filters, any preconceived ideas and instead I become an "empty vessel", where I allow myself to view my client's life through their eyes, so that I am able to notice their perceptions, thought patterns and beliefs.

I also create a sacred physical space, in which both my client and I are safe. Before any session I place the intention of being there fully for my client in order to help facilitate the deepest healing possible for them, so that they are able to connect with their own inner wisdom, love and divinity. I say a prayer, stating this intent. A prayer such as, "Dear _____ [Great Spirit, Higher Self, God, whatever you want to call this intelligence]. Please fill my mind, heart and body with your light and love. Let me see this person through your eyes. Let me see the divine beauty that shines within his/her heart and Soul. Let my thoughts be filled with light. Let my words be filled with wisdom, compassion, clarity and truth. Let my actions be guided by divine love. Let me be the way you would have me be. Please help me facilitate the best coaching session possible for my client so he/she gets the learnings, insights and wisdom he/she needs so he/she can heal this fully now. Let your loving wisdom guide me at all times. And so it is."

Then I imagine I create a sacred chamber, like a healing, nurturing sanctuary, in the room I am working in and I seal this space from any outside disturbance. I do this by imagining a bubble around this room – a bubble of light and healing.

During the session I go into such a deep state of rapport with my client that I start to notice how they experience life through their filters. This allows me to also know instinctively where it is I need to go in order to help them the most. As I am doing this, my clients feel completely accepted by me, so they start to open up. They trust me and together we start on a journey deep inside my client's Unconscious Mind, a journey deep inside the darkest corners of their mind, to their inner shadows, so that we can start to identify the deep inner-thought patterns that are now causing the problem in their life, which is the reason why they have come to me in the first place.

When you can be this way with people, just watch and see what happens. They start to open up, they dare to be vulnerable. Be a safe haven for people and you will build rapport and gain their confidence.

I always have an Unconscious Mind filter in place to stop me from absorbing my client's inner values, beliefs and negativity. Then after the session I let it all go and I cleanse myself by taking a shower and visualizing any negativity being washed away. I also mentally shower myself with light, internally and externally, before I leave the room, as well as cutting all the cords with my client, then throwing these cords on the imaginary healing fire, and seeing how the fire cleanses it all away (see Higher-Self Healing, pages 195–9). It only takes a few minutes and it helps enormously as it stops me from bringing my work home.

Chapter 18
In-depth Information on the Transformational Break-Through Healing Session

Questioning

A Transformational Break-Through Session usually takes around eight hours to complete, sometimes more, sometimes less, depending on how quickly you work as a coach and, more importantly, what kind of rapport your client has with their Unconscious Mind. Obviously, some clients come with really deep-seated problems (such as severe depression and suicidal thoughts) and they can, at times, take longer.

As a rough guide you should spend between 30 and 35 per cent of your session doing the questioning, as it is here you diagnose the root structures of the problem. Then the rest of the time is the intervention, which is when the problem structures are released. This is when the real healing and transformation take place. You can divide the Break-Through Session into two parts – the questioning and the intervention. I suggest you do not divide the intervention, as it is better to keep going once you start releasing the problem structures. If you have to divide the intervention, then keep the sessions close together. Doing the whole Break-Through Session in one go can be tiring, both for you and for your client. I used to always do them in one day, as that is how I was trained, but I would feel exhausted for days afterward. Then one day I was treating a young man and he fell asleep during the intervention. I had to wake him up, give him strong coffee and walk around with him outside. Since then I have divided the session into questioning and intervention.

I would also recommend that you work without time restraints, as it is impossible to know how responsive a particular client is going to be. This means that I never book another client in after my Break-Through client on the same day and I often see the Break-Through clients in the afternoon, leaving the morning free to see other clients and patients.

Pre-frame during the questioning session

Your client comes in with a problem and you start by explaining the Conscious Mind and Unconscious Mind, Cause and Effect, perception is projection (see Spiritual Presuppositions, pages 24–5), our Inner Screening System (you check values after your intervention to make sure the client's inner screening system has changed), and how the body and mind are linked. Then you take them through the questions below:

Break-Through questions for coaches

"Why are you here? Why else? Why else?" I usually spend a fair bit of time on this question so that I can get the metaphor of the presenting problem and how it is linked to the client's past. I am like a spider weaving a web around the client's problem and I elicit various Problem Strategies, making sure I elicit the main deep problems, not the minor ones. During one training, one student got so carried away that she identified 13 Problem Strategies in her client. Most of these were variations on the three major ones, so she only needed to have done the three main Problem Strategies. Be selective and keep digging for the main Problem Strategies. I might also identify various Parts Conflicts, Limiting Beliefs and so on. I might spend from 30 minutes up to an hour and a half on this question. Then I move on to the next question.

- "If I had a magic wand, waved it in the air and your problem completely disappeared, now, for good, how would you know that it had gone? What would you feel, see, hear, think, notice?" (Elicits the Solution Strategy. If you want, you can also ask for colours, as this will "juice up" the submodalities.)
- "When do you do your problem?" (If your client is a bit confused and wonders which one you mean, just tell them, "You know, the one you came in with." Lump all the "little" problems together, as even

though you are diagnosing lots of different structures, lots of different Problem Strategies, Parts Conflicts and Limiting Beliefs, you are still dealing mainly with one Problem Inner Screening System).

- "How do you know it is time to do it?"
- "When don't you do it?"
- "How long have you had this problem?"
- "What have you done about it so far?"
- "Was there ever a time when you did not experience your problem?"
- "Describe what happened the very first time you experienced this problem."
- "Is there a relationship between that first event and the problem as it is now?"
- "What has happened since that first event?"
- "When you think of your problem, what emotions do you feel, and where in your body do you feel them?" (You release this later with a Somato-Emotional Drop Down Through.)
- "Tell me about your childhood in relation to this problem."
- "Is there a connection between your problem and your relationship with your mother, father, siblings and any other key figure during your childhood?" (Ask about each of them all separately.)
- "Ask your Unconscious Mind, what is the purpose of having this problem in your life and when did you decide to create it?"
- "If there was anything your Unconscious Mind might want you to pay attention to, such that if you were to pay attention to it your problem would completely disappear, what would it be?"
- "Is there anything your Unconscious Mind wants you to know and learn, so that when you know and learn it, it would make your problem disappear?"
- "What are you pretending not to know by having your problem in your life?"
- "Look at what the possible outcome would be when you change this negative situation into a positive one and compare that with what would happen if you allowed the problem to stay the same. Look ahead one year from now and notice the difference. Five years from now. Ten years from now. Do you want the problem to change?"

(They need to say "Yes" here. If not, reframe, reframe, reframe until they say "Yes". If they do not say "Yes", send them home!)

It is important that you as a coach find out the Secondary Gain (the rewards the client is receiving from having their problem), so that you are aware of how attached the client is to having the problem and so that you make sure the Positive Learnings and Insights you get later during the intervention are strong enough to release the Secondary Gain). Ask the following questions:

- "What is this problem preventing you from doing, which if this problem disappeared, you'd have to do?"
- "What is it you are not doing because this problem is in your life?"
- "What is it that you are doing, which you enjoy doing, that you won't be able to do when your problem disappears?"
- "What is it that you are not doing, that you don't want to do, that you will have to do when your problem disappears?"

Finding the monster fish

During this questioning session, you can ask, "So if you were to look at yourself over there, what is it that you believe about yourself that has caused you to have this problem? What is it that you are that has caused you to create this problem?"

If your client ever articulates a Limiting Belief, which has the word "not" in it, such as "I am not good enough", then ask:

1. "So what are you that is causing you to believe you are not good enough?"
2. "What is it that you believe about yourself that is causing you to believe you are not good enough?"

These questions will give you some very deep Limiting Beliefs. Then you write them all down on a list and you ask your client to tell you which of them is the strongest one, which if it disappeared, all the others would go, too. Then you do the same with the second strongest one and the third, so you get at least the top three Limiting Beliefs. Now ask your client the following questions:

- "Ask your Unconscious Mind if it is totally willing to assist and support us in you having an undeniable experience of having this problem disappearing here during our session together." You have to get a "Yes" from your client, as otherwise you cannot release the problem. If you get a "No", you have to reframe, reframe, reframe until you get a "Yes". If you still do not get a "Yes", you have to tell the client that she is not ready for this work and that when she is ready, she is more than welcome to come back. But until then, you cannot work with her. Then you send the client home.

- "How do you know someone has done a good job? Do you have to see them do it, hear them doing it, experience them doing it, or analyze them doing it?" Gives you the client's convincer (the part inside the Unconscious Mind that decides whether we are convinced something has worked or not – this comes under Metaprogrammes, which are not covered in this book), so you know how your client knows whether something works or not. Use this during the coaching session to fill up their convincer. For example, if the client has to see someone doing a good job to know they have done the job well, you can say to your client during the session, "As you now look at yourself, can you see how much you have changed now? Can you see how you are empowered with all your Positive Learnings and Insights?"

- "How often does someone have to demonstrate competence to you before you are convinced they are good at what they do? Immediately, a certain number of times, over a certain period of time or never?" Once you know the answer to this one, you will use it to fill up their convincer during Higher-Self Healing. So, for example, say they have a three-times convincer (this means they need to experience something three times before their inner convincer is convinced!), then as they float back from the event to now, you get them to notice at least three events in the past and fill those events now with all their Positive Learnings and Insights and ask them to notice how that heals and transforms those events. And if their convincer was a period of time, for example three months, then you use that when you ask them to float out into the future, three months from now, and there ask them to notice how much they have changed now, enriched with all their Positive Learnings and Insights. This fills up their convincer.

- "What was the last thing you said to yourself before you got out of bed this morning?" This gives you the Auditory Digital portion of their motivation strategy and you then use this back to them. For example, if the last thing they said to themselves just before they got out of bed was, "It's time to get up", you can use this by saying: "It's time to change now", "It's time you heal this now".
- Values elicitation of the main area they are working with. Put them in order and elicit the positive and negative per cent on all the values. *Do not change anything or comment on anything here.*

The different areas for values elicitation (the client chooses one):
- Family
- Relationships
- Work/being of service
- Health and well-being
- Personal development
- Spiritual development

Intervention

Once you have gone through the questions with your client, you will transfer everything you have found on to an Intervention Document, structured like this one.

Intervention Document
Unconscious Mind signals – "Yes" / "No"

Higher-Self Healing to release:
1. Problem Strategy/Strategies

   Write down all the Problem Strategies you have found. But remember to only elicit the main problems (the main big monster fish and not just lots of little ones).
2. Negative Emotions

   Write down all the Negative Emotions you have found.

   As you release the Problem Strategies you have probably released some of these Negative Emotions, too, so if you think this has happened, then before releasing a Negative Emotion you think might have gone, ask them, "Is this _____ [specific Negative Emotion] still there for you, or has it now gone?"

You then calibrate to see whether it is there or not by using the client's Unconscious Mind's "Yes" and "No" signals.

3. Limiting Beliefs

You first write down the top three Limiting Beliefs, and you always release the top one.

You write down all the Limiting Beliefs you have found during the questioning session. Remember you cannot release a Limiting Belief which has a "not" in it.

Some Limiting Beliefs will have been released by you having done the work on Problem Strategies and Negative Emotions, so just as you did for Negative Emotions, check first for each Limiting Belief whether it is still there or whether it has now gone.

Healing with the Highest Intention Reframe of problem

Always do this on the main problems found.

Anchor

Use a Collapse Anchor (see pages 92–4) if needed. Also teach Resource Anchor (see pages 89–91) if needed.

Parts Integration (if needed)

Always write down all the Parts Conflicts you have identified. By the time you do the Parts Integration exercise many Parts Conflicts will have healed through the previous work. Before you release a Parts Conflict here ask, "So how is that a problem now? How is that a conflict?"

If they say that it is not a problem any more and you calibrate that this is correct, then you know you do not need to do a Parts Integration. If they say it is still there, and/or you calibrate it is still there, then you release it.

Submodalities

Do this if it is needed. It can at times be useful to do Mapping Across of Problem State to Solution State. So here elicit all the submodalities of the Problem State (so "As you think of your problem, do you have a picture?"), and then of the Solution State ("If I had a magic wand and waved it in the air, so this problem would be gone now, how would you know it has gone? What would you see, feel, hear, notice, say to yourself? As you think of that, do you have a picture?"). Then do contrasting analysis of these two states, and then map the Problem State into the submodalities of the Solution State. (See Submodalities, pages 64–85).

Somato-Emotional Drop Down Through on a body part associated with the problem

This also becomes a checkpoint for the coach, since if the problem has fully gone, the client will very quickly drop into a positive inner essence. (Do not be surprised if they immediately come to a Positive Layer; that is quite normal at the end of a Break-Through Session.) If there is still work to do, then you are able to get to it from a different angle with this exercise. Drop Down Through gives us a metaphor of how that client relates to their problem in their lives.

Forgiveness Exercise (and Perceptual Positions if needed)

Write down the names of all the people they need to do this with, including their parents, siblings and present family, as well as other key figures.

Goal-setting

Setting goals is important to help give the Unconscious Mind a direction. Make sure the goals are stated in the positive and will help to cement the learnings the client's Unconscious Mind has given during the session.

Re-checking of Values in the same area they did before

All values have to be 100 per cent positive before you allow the client to go home. If a value is not 100 per cent positive, then ask them, "As you are now, within yourself in your thoughts, after our having done all this work together, is there anything, in your thoughts, that could stop you from moving with 100 per cent positivity toward creating this in your life now?"

When I ask clients this they realize that, as they are now in their thoughts, there is nothing that can stop them moving forward toward creating this value in their lives. So I then ask, "Great, so how much positive energy do you feel in association with this value now, as you are in your thoughts right now?"

Final Meditation, including meeting the Future You and the Solution Strategy

This will help you to make sure that the client runs their Solution Strategy as they go home. What can also be nice to do is to take them straight into meeting their Authentic Self and you finish the session with them writing a letter from their Authentic Self about how they can be, what they can do and what that will allow them to have in their life.

Additional information about Higher-Self Healing

When you are working with a client, you can use the downloadable script for Higher-Self Healing as mentioned previously (see page 193). You can also use some variations to that script, which are outlined below.

When you do this exercise, your client may go to any event in the past. This may be in childhood, in the womb or even before that. If they do go to a past life, or to an event that happened to one of their parents or was inherited down the generations, then see this as a metaphor that their Unconscious Mind is presenting them with, in order for them to get the insights, learnings and wisdom they need to release this.

To get the event your client needs to work with, you can use one of the following options:

Option A

- "Ask your Unconscious Mind when was the first time you felt this _____ [Problem Strategy, Negative Emotion, Limiting Belief]. Your Unconscious Mind is very wise and knows everything that has ever happened to you. Just trust it to guide you to the right event and allow your Unconscious Mind to float you up in the air, all the way back into the past where you first felt this _____ [Problem Strategy,

Negative Emotion, Limiting Belief], or to the event your Unconscious Mind feels is the best one for you to work with today so you can get the Learnings you need. Let me know when you are there."

Option B

- "I would now like to ask your Unconscious Mind:
  'When was the very first time you felt this _____ [Problem Strategy, Negative Emotion, Limiting Belief], the event, which when released will heal this fully? If you were to know, was it before, during or after your birth?'" (Wait until you get an answer.)
- If "after" ask, "If you were to know, how old were you?"
- If "before" ask, "Was it in the womb or before that?"
- If "in the womb" ask, "If you were to know, how old were you?"
- If "before" ask, "Was it at the time of conception, in a past life or did you inherit it from your parents?"
- If "in a past life" ask, "If you were to know, how many lifetimes ago?"
- If "from my parents" ask, "From which side (give them time to answer) and how many generations ago?"

During Step 5 of Higher Self-Healing (see page 196):

After you have done the Forgiveness Exercise, you can also do Perceptual Positions. You only do this if you feel you need more leverage in order for your client to be able to forgive the people involved in the event. Use your calibration to know when and when not. Usually I do not need to use it, but sometimes a client is really stuck and needs more insights in order to be able to forgive and let go.

Trouble-shooting for Higher-Self Healing

1. What do I do if my client can't see a memory?

Some people cannot see what is going on in the event – that is fine. Their Unconscious Mind knows what is going on; it is just that the Unconscious Mind will not let the Conscious Mind know what it is. The main aspect that releases the negative feelings associated with the event are the Positive Learnings, Insights and Wisdom, so once you have got these you just ask your client to float down inside the event (even if they cannot see what is going on) and notice that the Negative Emotions have gone now. You probably cannot take the client through the Forgiveness Exercise or Perceptual Positions.

2. **If they can't see the memory, how do I know they are at the right event?**

First ask their Unconscious Mind. If that does not work, then get them to float inside the event first and then float above and before the event. If the Negative Emotion disappears when they float above and before the event, but is stronger when they are at the event, then they are at an event that contained lots of Negative Emotion for them.

3. **What do I do if they go to a "weird" memory?**

Remember, the event is just a metaphor, so at times a client may go to a metaphor that you know is not real, but it gives the client a chance to work out the pattern of the problem so that they can get the Positive Learnings needed to heal the problem. Clients have been known to go to varied metaphors such as: a black horse, an abandoned castle, a squid, a cave with monkeys, a snake pit and so on. This "event" has never happened, but it represented the problem perfectly and was what the client needed to work with to shift and heal the problem.

4. **What do I do if the client is alone in the event?**

You ask for the Positive Learnings, Insights and Wisdom from the event and, if needed, do a Forgiveness Exercise for the younger aspect of themselves in the event – use the camp fire and so on.

5. **What do I do if the client goes back to an event that does not involve them (such as an event inherited through their parents)?**

Do the same as for Step 4, asking for Positive Learnings, Forgiveness Exercise and the camp fire. Just see the event as a metaphor.

6. **What do I do if the event is extremely traumatic?**

You take them straight out of it and up high to the sacred mountain. You can also tell them to scoop up the younger version of themselves in that event, so that part of them feels safe. You may need to do a phobia cure (a modified version is outlined below) while being up in a third position above the event (such as on the mountain or on a cloud in the sky). This is what I do:

a) Get them to be above the event (on a mountain top or a cloud) and see the event way down there. They need to see it as a movie on a movie screen and make a mark in the movie, with an x, when they feel *safe at the beginning* and with another x when they realize they are *safe at the end*.

b) Let the movie run forward in black and white from where the client was safe at the beginning to when they realized they were safe again (they are still sitting up on the mountain or on a cloud, and the movie screen is way, way down there, so they are disassociated from the event).

c) White out or black out the movie when it comes to an end. If they want to, they can also white out or black out the area where the phobia/emotional response was created.

d) Then ask them to run the movie backward in colour from the end when they were safe, to the beginning when they were safe, while singing a silly song to themselves. Repeat Steps 2 to 4 until the Negative Emotion has completely gone.

I sometimes combine this with the Forgiveness Exercise (see pages 209–11), if the response is in relation to an event involving another person, and I then get them to cut the cords and place them all in a cleansing fire. This has proven very effective when, for example, someone has gone back to an event where they were abused. If they go back to an event like this or they experienced something horrific, I also get them to quickly scoop up the younger version of themselves and take the younger self up to above and before the event, where they are safe, and from this safe place they can then watch the movie of the event together. You keep repeating the words "safe, safe, safe", which will sink into your client's Unconscious Mind, so all they hear is "safe", and it is then easier for them to release the Negative Emotions they have associated with the event.

You can also use the column of fire (from the healing fire up on the sacred mountain, as outlined in the Higher-Self Healing Process on page 196) and send it back and forth, back and forth, from the beginning of the event when they were safe to the end of the event when they were safe, and this column of fire just burns away any old negativity, until all that is left is a healing, peaceful light. A phobic response is just a very intense, extremely fearful response.

7. **What do I do if they go back to a past life and I don't believe in past lives or my client does not believe in past lives?**

   Just see the event as a metaphor the Unconscious Mind is presenting to the client; a metaphor in which the Positive Learnings that are needed for this wound to heal now are present. The event is never the important part, whereas the learnings are. The past is gone and the drama of it will never heal us; only the Positive Learnings can. Once we get the Positive Learnings, Insights and Wisdom present in the traumatic event, whenever the event happened, we can let it go and move forward. Some people find it easier to go back to something that is just being seen as a metaphor, because they cannot relate it to an event in this lifetime, and as long as they get the learnings they need so that they are able to release the wound, then that is all that matters.

8. **What do I do if the client goes back to an event where another person is abusing them?**

   You take them straight out of the event and fly above it, scooping the younger person up with them to the sacred mountain, and do not invite the abuser up to the mountain. You also avoid doing Perceptual Positions. I usually do the Forgiveness Exercise only, cut the cords, and of course also use the cleansing fire, as it is a great transformative agent for letting go of the past.

9. **What do I do if my client is terrified about going back into the past and about feeling emotions?**

   This has only happened to me once and I used Perceptual Positions for all the emotions. I got the client to feel a particular emotion, say anger, then asked him, "So who do you most often feel this anger is connected to?" Then we did Perceptual Positions with that person.

   We released all the Negative Emotions this way, and he still got the results he needed. I just skipped the Higher-Self Healing for releasing Problem Strategies, Negative Emotions and Limiting Beliefs. He could still do all the other processes, such as Parts Integration, Somato-Emotional Drop Down Through, submodalities of Mapping Across of Problem State to Solution State and so on. Just be flexible and willing to try new approaches.

10. **What do I do if the Positive Learnings are not that positive?**

Keep asking the client, "What other Positive Learnings are there?" If that is not enough, you can ask them to float even higher, to an even higher mountain top and they then again invite their most evolved, Wise Self, or their Higher Conscious Mind, or their spirit, or their soul (use words that are in alignment with your client's Model of the World – never force your Model of the World on them), and if they could ask this wise being now what the Positive Learnings are for them so that they can heal this event now, what would those Positive Learnings be?

Doing this tends to get the client to access insights and wisdom from a Higher Logical Level than they were able to access previously. You are, in effect, taking them up to a very high third position, to a position of divine wisdom. Usually, though, this is not necessary as you have already taken your client up to a sacred mountain, but if you are working with a client who has difficulty being spiritually stretched, then just get them to go higher and higher, to an even more sacred place, high, high up. By doing this, her Unconscious Mind will start to get the message!

An effective technique for a client who gives a Positive Learning in the form of a negative, such as, "I don't have to be stressed about this", is to ask in reply, "So what can you be instead?" This will guide your client to discover what she can do instead of being stressed and it will help her find the Positive Learning.

11. **What do I do if my client just cannot find an event?**

This is very rare, but if it does happen, I just get the client to float up to the sacred mountain top and sit up there, by the healing fire, and invite their Wise Higher Self to be up there with them. And by sitting so high up above their life, they can now see clearly all the times when they went into the pattern of _____ [Problem Strategy, Negative Emotion, Limiting Belief – whatever you are working on]. Which people do they feel and which can they see, who are linked with this? Then you invite these people also to be up here with them on the mountain top. Do the Forgiveness Exercise with all of them (and cut any negative cords), including also from the younger version of the client, ask the Wise Higher Self for all the Positive Learnings, cut the cords with all the times that the client has gone into this pattern, throw it all on the healing fire, get the fire to cleanse it all away until it is all gone and a new positive energy is rising from the fire. Ask the client to breathe it in and then to float back from the mountain over her life, sprinkling down all her Positive Insights and Learnings and gifts from the fire into her life all the way back to now, and then you also take this out into the future.

On the very rare occasion you have a client who cannot even do the above, I would use the following:

- Perceptual Positions (find the people they feel are linked with their problem and do Perceptual Positions with each and every one).
- Mapping Across (on all negative states and map them, one by one, across to a positive state).
- Collapse Anchors (on all negative states and triggers).

What to do after you have completed Higher-Self Healing

Once you have finished with all the Problem Strategies, Negative Emotions and Limiting Beliefs, you do Healing with the Highest Intention Reframe (see pages 95–101) on the presenting problem, Collapse Anchoring if needed (usually not needed), submodalities if needed (usually not needed, but if you do it, just do it from Problem State to Solution State), Parts Integration if needed (at times it is needed, but you have to check first whether the Parts Conflict is still there, by asking: "So how is that a problem now?"; if it is not a problem any more, then you do not do the Parts Conflict process) and Somato-Emotional Drop Down Through on the body area or areas where the problem was felt.

Then you move into forgiveness (take the client through this process in relation to their parents, siblings, and also if they have a partner and children). Remember to work really quickly here. The whole exercise should only take between five and 10 minutes as the client has already practised so much forgiveness during the Higher-Self Healing process. Why you do it again here is that you are closing the wound you have initially opened, so you are making sure your client is fully whole before they leave you. After that you carry out goal-setting, and then you re-check the values.

After re-checking values you then take the client through the final meditation, where they meet the Future You and their Authentic Self.

We will now cover values and the final meditation in more detail than previously. The other processes have already been outlined.

Re-checking values

After goals re-check the values and make sure they are all 100 per cent positive. Do not let the client go home until they are all 100 per cent positive. Tell them that, too (this is a double-bind, since if they want to go home they have to change!). If the values are 100 per cent positive this is a great convincer for them, and also one way that you can make sure your work is completed. Read the section in Part 5 (see pages 216–17) in which the Angel Coach talks about re-checking values (what you say to a client). This will help you to make sure the values are all 100 per cent positive.

If the values are not 100 per cent positive

If they are not 100 per cent positive (and that is *really* rare), you have to use reframes to get the client to realize the consequence of that choice, because it is all in their thoughts and they are choosing their thoughts. Let me give you an example:

One client was working on relationships and her values before the intervention had been, among many others, love and trust. They had been 90 per cent negative.

After the intervention, she still had love and trust as her top two values. The following then took place:

Coach: "Why is love important to you now?"

Client: "Because that is what we are."

Coach: "Great, so how much is that then a positive value for you?"

Client: "80 per cent."

Coach: "OK, so as you are now in your thoughts, is there anything that could be stopping you from moving toward creating love in your relationship?"

Client: "No."

Coach: "Great, so how much is that then a positive value for you, in that you have positive energy in moving toward creating love in your relationship?"

Client: "90 per cent."

Coach: "OK, so as you are now, is there anything that could be stopping you from moving toward creating love in your relationship?"

Client: "Well, I want my partner to be more loving toward me."

Coach: "OK, so you want your partner to be more loving toward you, so therefore you are withholding 10 per cent of positive energy of love toward your partner. Now as soon as we withhold love from our partner in our thoughts, imagine what will happen with that 10 per cent over time? It will increase. So for what purpose would you choose to do that in your thoughts? For what purpose would you do that to your relationship?"

Client: "Oh, I never thought about it in that way. Well, there is no purpose. I want us to be happy together."

Coach: "Great, so how much is that then a positive value for you *as you are in your thoughts now*?"

Client: "Oh, it is 100 per cent," she said with a great smile of relief.

Coach: "OK, so why is trust important to you now?"

Client: "Because trust is what cements you together."

Coach: "Great. So how much is that a positive value for you?"

Client: "Oh, it is 90 per cent."

Coach: "OK, so as you are now in your thoughts, is there anything that could be stopping you from moving toward creating trust in your relationship?"

Client: "I just want to have proof first that I can trust my partner."

Coach: "OK, so for what purpose would you withhold trust from your partner? What do you think will happen with the trust between you if you now, in your thoughts, are withholding 10 per cent of trust from your partner? Everything starts with our thoughts, so in order for you to have external proof, you first have to change your thinking, since your thoughts create your reality and you know that, don't you? (Client nods at this point – she is fully aware of this). So for what purpose would you choose to plant a seed of non-trust in your relationship?"

Client: "No purpose. That is just stupid. I don't know what I was thinking."

Coach: "Great. So as you now think about trust, how much is that now a positive value for you?"

Client: "100 per cent."

The client was visibly relieved and happy by this point and from then on all her other values were 100 per cent positive. It was particularly difficult to get her to realize that she had changed in her thoughts and that her thoughts had indeed changed *independently* of her partner. The only person we can change is ourselves and we start by changing our *thinking*. I am happy to report, though, that this client is now very, very happy with her partner.

Final Meditation

In the final mediation you want your client to relax fully, connecting with the peace and stillness within them, and then you feed back their Solution Strategy to them, as well as all the major Positive Learnings their Unconscious Mind has communicated to them during the session.

A suggested example of a Final Meditation

"Close your eyes and feel how you sink into your inner stillness. Feel whether there is any tension in your body. Increase that tension as you breathe in and as you breathe out let that tension go (say this following the same pace as your client's in- and out-breaths). Do this now with another area of your body that you feel is tense. So increase that tension as you breathe in and as you breathe out just let that tension go.

"Now float with your awareness inside your mind. Feel whether there is any tension in your mind, increase that tension as you breathe in and as you breathe out just let that tension go. Now go to another area of your mind that you feel is tense. Breathe in as you increase that tension and, as you breathe out, just let that tension go.

"Just focus on your breathing, breathing in ... and out, sinking deeper and deeper into the stillness within you and as you are sitting here, breathing in and out, listening to me, relaxing more and more, you can just imagine how you are opening up the top of your head, drawing in a universal white light through the top of your head and every time you breathe in, you breathe in this white light, and every time you breathe out, you breathe out everything you no longer need and you see it leave you as grey smoke. Breathing in the light ... breathing out grey smoke ... breathing in light, filling your whole mind and body with light ... breathing out everything you no longer need. Just keep breathing in this light, filling every cell of your body and mind with light, and as you do, thank yourself for having done this work on yourself.

"Imagine now floating up again to that beautiful, sacred mountain. When you reach the top you can see the Future You coming toward you to greet you. Notice what the Future You looks like and what qualities they have. Ask the Future You any questions you have and wait for the answers. They will come, as words, feelings or images.

"Your Future You has a message for you. This message is a gift to you, a positive message, which will help you on your journey through life. Make sure you get this message. (Write down this message for your client.)

"Now feel yourself merge with the Future You, so that you fully integrate all the knowledge, wisdom and compassion your Future You has.

"Look at the view from this mountain. From one side of this mountain you can see your old life, the way you used to be, and on the other side of the mountain you can see your new life, the life you now can live enriched with all your learnings, insights and wisdom. It is your choice as to which path you want to go down – into your old life or into your new life. Choose wisely. So which path are you going to choose?" (Allow time for an answer and your client should answer, "Into my new life.")

You then say, "That's great! You have done so well and remember all the Positive Learnings your Unconscious Mind and Wise Higher Self have communicated to you, _____ [here tell them all the major Positive Learnings] and all the Positive Resources and gifts your inner wisdom has given you of _____ [here tell them the resources and gifts they have been given during the session]. Feel how all of these are now integrating within you, within the very core of you and how you are _____ [here feed back their Solution Strategy, which you found during your Break-Through questioning].

251

"Now imagine that all these Positive Resources, gifts and insights are colours, which colours would they be?" (Ask your client to tell you which colours they are.)

"Now let your whole body and mind become filled with these positive colours of _____ [repeat the colours your client gave you], and let these colours now spin faster and faster inside your body, so you are filled with happy, sparkling colours. Imagine now you have in your hands a sacred hosepipe and you let these colours float inside it, and as you sit up here on this sacred mountain, you are so high, high up that you can see your whole life down there, the whole timeline of your past, the now and the future. Now spin these colours faster and faster and let these positive colours, resources, insights and wisdom float inside this hosepipe and flow into your past, like a healing rain, cleansing your past so it becomes filled with _____ [the colours your client gave you] and continue to send these colours into your whole past until it is sparkling, then do the same now with the present moment filling it with _____ [the colours your client gave you] and then turn this hosepipe to your future and fill your future with these positive colours of _____ [the colours your client gave you], so that your future becomes filled with all your Positive Learnings and Insights of _____ [learnings, insights, resources and gifts your client has stated previously], so that your whole future becomes filled with light, filled with amazing colours and it is positively sparkling and shining.

"As you are doing this, filling every cell of your body, every moment of your life, all the way out into eternity, then come back with your awareness into the now and see in front of you an amazingly beautiful being. You realize this being is your own Authentic Self. See the light and wisdom that shines deep within your Authentic Self's eyes. See the beauty that radiates all around your Authentic Self. See which positive qualities your Authentic Self has. Feel the positive energy coming from your Authentic Self and allow yourself to be filled with this positive energy.

"Now ask your Authentic Self what your life purpose is? [Ask your client to tell you what the answer is.] Which unique, spiritual [only use the word "spiritual" if your client is open to that terminology] gifts do you have to share with the world? [Give the client time to answer.] How can you best do that? [Give the client time to answer.]

"Then feel yourself merge with your Authentic Self, so that you become one. Feel this integration take place and know how everything you have done during this session, all the insights you have had, all the learnings, have allowed you to now live your life as your Authentic Self, and then when you have fully integrated all of this, you will soon, slowly, slowly, open your eyes and as your Authentic Self you will in a moment write a letter to yourself, advising yourself on what you need to do to live your life to the full. What action do you need to take? What do you need to change? What do you need to let go of? What do you need to embrace? What steps do you need to take? What qualities do you need to cultivate and what do you need to focus on in order to create an authentic life filled with happiness and wisdom? So when you are fully ready to embrace your Authentic Self's wisdom, come back into this present moment and into your life fully, and when you are ready to live your life being filled with your divine wisdom, insights and resources, then and only then can you open your eyes.

"Please write this letter now in complete silence. This letter is only for you. It is a sacred, private letter from your most Authentic Self to you."

Chapter 19
Before and After a Transformational Break-Through Healing Session

Before you see a client

Before you see a client, interview them over the phone (or by email) to make sure they are willing to take responsibility for their lives, and also to see if they are suitable for you to work with. Also before you agree to take them on, ask them to answer the following questions in writing:

1. If you could have anything from your session, what would it be?
2. What have you got in your life that you no longer want?
3. What have you not got in your life that you now want?
4. Write a short life history including both positive and negative events.
5. What patterns have you noticed occurring in your life?

This constitutes the first task you give your client, but if they cannot be bothered to answer these questions, I would urge you not to work with them. You need your client to be willing to work with you and to do *whatever it takes* to shift the problem.

Once you have received the answers and you are satisfied that you can work with this client, then you can book the client in for a Break-Through Session. You can do the session in one day, or divide it into two sessions (to a maximum of three sessions). I usually divide it into two sessions, the first being the questioning and the second the intervention.

Deposit, insurance and letter from a medical practitioner

Always take a deposit if you are booking someone in for a Break-Through Healing Session, and if the client does not turn up they lose their deposit. I would recommend the deposit being between 30 and 50 per cent of the total cost of the session.

Always take out insurance and never treat anyone without insurance.

If your client is suffering from depression or panic attacks, or you feel you would like support from their family doctor or psychotherapist, then always ask for a letter from them stating that the client is suitable for coaching. *Never* see the client until you have received this letter.

Coaching contract, taking notes, keeping notes, seeing children

Always take out a contract with your client before you start the first session. (You will find a sample on page 256.)

Also remember that you have to take notes, which are legal documents. They must be kept for seven years for adult clients and for 10 years for child clients. You must keep these documents in a safe place and as these notes and your sessions are confidential, you cannot show them to anyone or make them available publicly.

Children under the age of 16 have to be accompanied by an adult. I usually ask the adult to sit outside the consultation room, with the door open, so that the parent can see that everything happening in the room is fine. This is actually to protect you, as a coach, from being sued for behaving in an unprofessional manner toward a minor.

Children are great to work with, as they respond really quickly. I have found you can work easily with children over the age of eight, but below that age it depends on their emotional and mental maturity. This means that I can never guarantee to the parents that NLP and coaching can be used with the child, but if the child is over the age of five years I am happy to meet the child and find out.

Sample Transformational NLP coaching contract

This agreement is between _____ (the client)

Date _____ Address _____

Postcode _____

and _____ (the coach)

I, the client fully understand:

- A coaching session in no way replaces diagnosis or advice from a medical doctor or a psychiatrist.
- I need to tell my coach before the session if I have a history of mental illness.
- The result of the coaching session is dependent upon my communication with my Unconscious Mind, which I am 100 per cent responsible for and my coach can only facilitate.
- The result of the coaching session is dependent upon me following the instructions that my coach gives me as she guides me through the processes of NLP and Transformational Coaching. The responsibility for making the processes work for me is solely mine as no one else can do it for me.
- The long-term result of this coaching session is 100 per cent dependent upon me following the tasks my coach sets me and following the advice my own Unconscious Mind has given me during this session. I also need to focus on what I want and take action to get me there.
- My coach is not a mind-reader and my coach cannot assist me in resolving issues I do not share with my coach.
- All sessions are recorded in a written format for future reference.

On this basis I agree to commit to working with my coach and I acknowledge that the cost of the session is _____ per hour/session. To secure my booking a non-refundable deposit of _____ is needed, which will be deducted from the final price. The length of the session is dependent upon the rapport between my Unconscious Mind and my Conscious Mind, a process only my coach can facilitate.

What not to treat

Coaches should be wary of treating major depression, severe panic attacks, severe health problems, severe eating disorders (anorexia and bulimia), severe mental and emotional problems, *unless they have previous experience of working with these conditions* and are qualified to do so.

For example, I would not see someone who is suffering from paranoid schizophrenia or acute manic depression (bipolar disorder), or psychosis, since I am not qualified to treat these conditions – and I am a trainer in NLP. Know your limitations. This is to make sure you are always safe and that the person you are working with is always safe with you. There are plenty of people out there who need help, so choose those that you can help the most. *Know your professional boundaries.*

When to refer someone

Remember that you do not have to treat someone just because they have come to see you. Over the years I have sent some people away, but I make sure I refer them to someone else.

Sometimes people are just not ready to change – if you detect this send them to someone else, such as another complementary practitioner, or back to their medical practitioner. You can stop a session with a client at any time; if you feel your client is not yet ready, or that the presenting problem is one that you are not equipped to help with. I have also, on occasion, when I have noticed a client not cooperating, told them that they either start cooperating or we finish the session there and then. So far, I have usually found that just highlighting to the client that they are playing a "game" of resisting change is all that is needed – and they then start to be more cooperative.

What not to say

Also remember that you can never say you can "cure" anything – that is illegal. You can only say you treat the symptoms of X, Y and Z, that you treat the person – never the illness itself. When someone comes to me with a physiological illness I always say that I can only help them release various stresses and strains within their body, mind and spirit connection, which will enable them to have more energy available, but how the body and mind chooses to use that extra available energy I cannot control. Hence I can never know if they will get better or not. I am only a facilitator. You can never heal anything – the person you are working with heals him/herself. It has absolutely nothing to do with you – you facilitate only.

After a Break-Through Healing Session

I always send a letter to the client after a Break-Through Healing Session, where I outline all the Positive Learnings, Insights and Wisdom communicated by the client's Unconscious Mind (only the positive ones – never any negative, so-called learnings), and Higher Self (only use the word Higher Self if your client is comfortable with that – otherwise just call it Wise Self). I also include in the letter important pointers for the client to remember, and I make sure these pointers are *positive*. I never tell the client which Problem Strategies, Limiting Beliefs and so on we have released, as that could instil them again. I focus only on the positive.

I also give them various exercises to do, and tasking, which will help to really deepen their new way of being, deepen the Solution Strategy now running in their lives.

Tasking

I often give tasks in between two sessions, which could be that the client meditates daily, or does the Forgiveness Exercise, or writes letters containing everything they feel angry, sad, anxious, worried, guilty and fearful about (and any other Negative Emotions diagnosed), and that they then burn these letters. I always calibrate what is most suitable for each individual client.

Conclusion for coaches

Transformational NLP use superb tools for facilitating deep healings. The more you have healed yourself, the more able you will be to pace and lead your client to a place where they can connect with the wholeness within.

Therefore it is important to continue to work on yourself, become aware of your own darkness and issues and take steps to release them, so that you can connect more fully with your divine light.

Transformational NLP is just a tool – it is the energy and intent behind the person using this tool that creates the difference. It is also important to remember that working on ourselves is a journey and a process so we have to refrain from thinking we are ever finished. There is always more to learn, more discoveries to be made, another level of wisdom to evolve to.

You can use Transformational NLP to enable others to awaken from the grip of their ego to the divine consciousness living inside them. Before you help to awaken others you have to awaken yourself. You can only help and awaken someone else to the same extent you have helped and awakened yourself, as you can only pace and lead someone to places you have been to yourself.

So be courageous! Be daring! Explore the exciting adventure that awaits you, as you dive into the depths of your mind, soul and spirit. You have within you untold riches, incredible resources, exquisite wisdom, and you find all of these when you journey into your Inner Self and connect with your Divine Self. As you find these riches, you are then able to take others on this incredible journey, too – this time you help them travel into their own inner world, where they too will find untold riches, amazing resources and exquisite wisdom inside of themselves. Your role as a coach is to facilitate the journey. A word of warning: *never do the journey for them and never tell them what these riches, resources and wisdom are.* In order for us to truly find our inner power and healing ability we have to find it ourselves. We have to make the journey there ourselves. It is like the two women I met on the mountain in Nepal (see chapter on Submodalities, pages 64–6). They discovered wonderful resources inside themselves: resources of strength, fun, courage and will-power, and they also became a source of inspiration to others who were blessed to meet them. You can be like their Nepalese guide to your clients. Show them the way and then let them make the journey themselves. You are just guiding them through the terrain, taking them through processes, creating a sacred space for them where they can go on this inner journey, this long trek, so your client can connect with the wisdom, power, happiness, love, energy and divine intelligence, which lives within each and every one of us.

So remember to let your clients do the actual work, and this also means you can never take credit for their results. You are just guiding them, facilitating the journey and it is the clients who find the resources within themselves to transform their lives.

Go on many treks within yourself, because the more used you become to the terrain, the more accustomed you will be to the higher altitude, the more skilled you will be as a guide and a coach. Just imagine all the amazing gifts you will bring through from these altitudes, gifts you can then share with others in your life.

And … above all, trekking is just such great fun!

Cissi Williams, Sigtuna, Sweden

Index